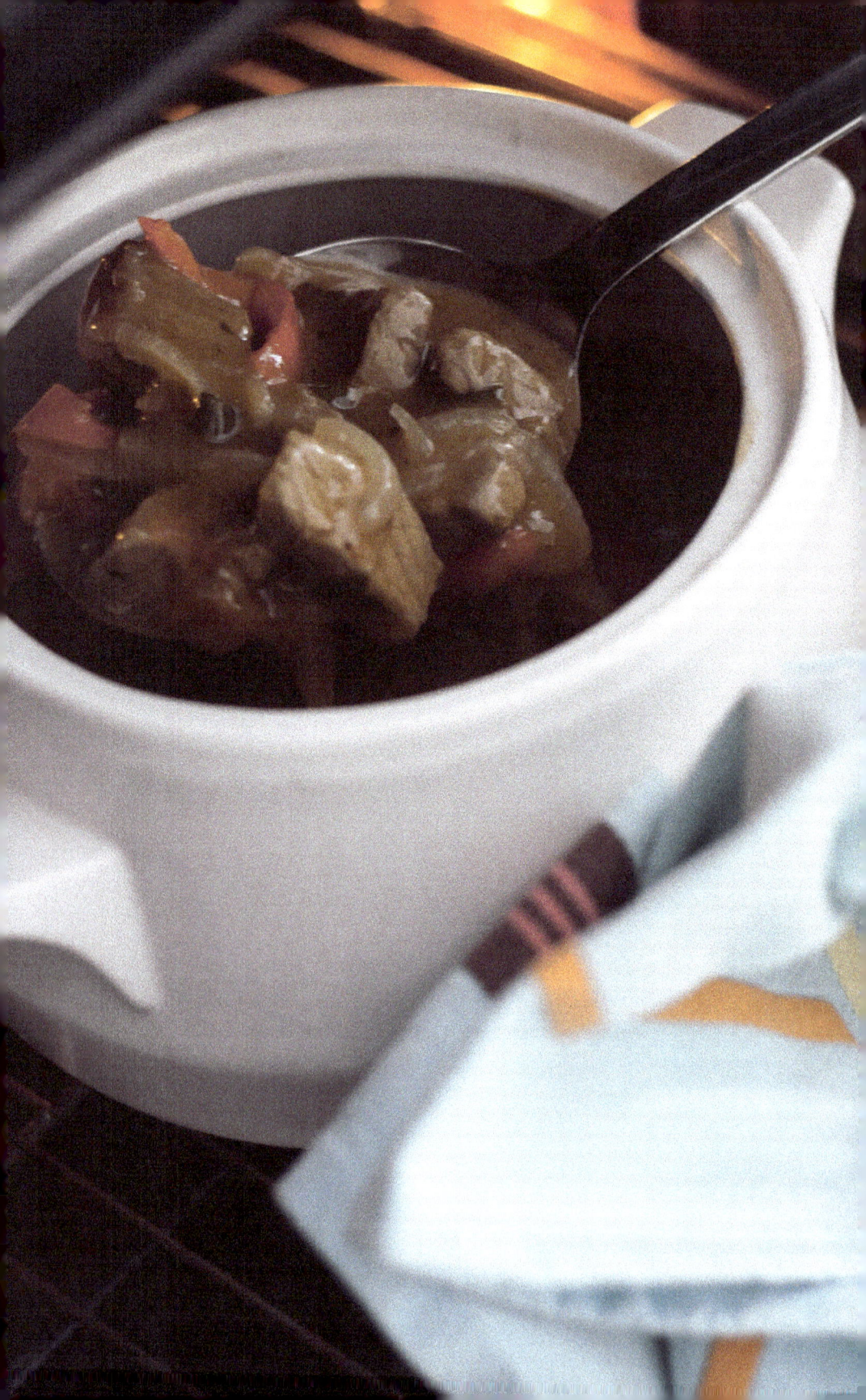

SIMPLE COOKING

for allergies & intolerances

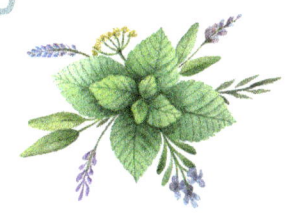

Cheree Heath
HH Dip D.N. & F.E.A.

Copyright © 2016

All rights reserved. No part of this publication may be reproduced, stored in a retrieval system or transmitted in any form by any means without the prior permission of the copyright owner. Enquiries should be made to the publisher.

Every effort has been made to ensure that this book is free from error or omissions. However, the Publisher, the Author, the Editor or their respective employees or agents, shall not accept responsibility for injury, loss or damage occasioned to any person acting or refraining from action as a result of material in this book whether or not such injury, loss or damage is in any way due to any negligent act or omission, breach of duty or default on the part of the Publisher, the Author, the Editor, or their respective employees or agents.

The Author, the Publisher, the Editor and their respective employees or agents do not accept any responsibility for the actions of any person - actions which are related in any way to information containted in this book.

The moral right of the author has been asserted.

National Library of Australia Cataloguing-in-Publication entry

Author: Heath, Cheree (HH Dip FN & DEA)

Title: Simple Cooking For Allegies & Intolerances

ISBN: 9780994412652

Subject: Cooking, Food, Allergies

Dewey Number: 641.5639

Images by agreement with photographers. Illustrations by Elena Medvedeva. The publisher has done its utmost to attribute the copyright holders of all the visual material used. If you nevertheless think that a copyright has been infringed, please contact the publisher.

Published by: Of The World Publishing
ACN 133 333 141
PO Box 8070
Bendigo South LPO VIC 3550

www.oftheworldbooks.com

CONTENTS

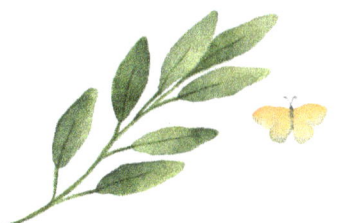

7
what
what foods have been avoided in this book

8
why
my journey and why I wrote this book

12
substitutes
common replacement foods to make cooking easier

14
adding flavour
using herbs and spices to make food taste fabulous

21
extras
23 herbed oil
25 garlic oil
27 basil oil
29 french dressing
31 mustard sauce
33 basil & anchovy sauce
35 chicken stock
37 vegetable stock

39
starters
41 avocado dip
43 red salmon dip
45 hommus dip
47 chunky vege & pork soup
49 chicken noodle soup
51 ministrone
53 spicy carrot soup
55 savoury scones
57 flat bread
59 fried rice

61
mains
63 stuffed rainbow trout
65 baked fish steaks
67 red salmon pie
69 chicken nuggets
71 chicken with lemon sauce
73 roast chicken
75 pork with mustard sauce
77 pork & garlic stir fry
79 french lamb casserole
81 crumbed lamb chops
83 irish stew
85 beef goulash
87 beef potato pie
89 vegetarian pasta
91 middle eastern stew

93
bbq
95 chicken kebabs
96 lamb kebabs
97 beef kebabs
99 asian pork
101 pepper steak
103 corn, mango & avocado salsa
105 tomato & cucumber salsa
107 fruit kebabs

109
desserts
111 golden pear pudding
113 peach mango bake
115 maple syrup dumplings
117 baked pear parcels
119 banana fritters
121 watermelon ice
123 banana & blueberry sorbet
125 mango gelato
127 berry tart
129 pomegranate jelly

131
eating out
living with allergies outside your own kitchen

133
index
an easy to find ingredient & recipe list

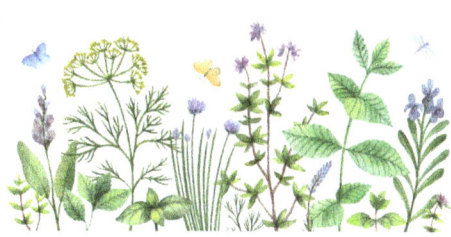

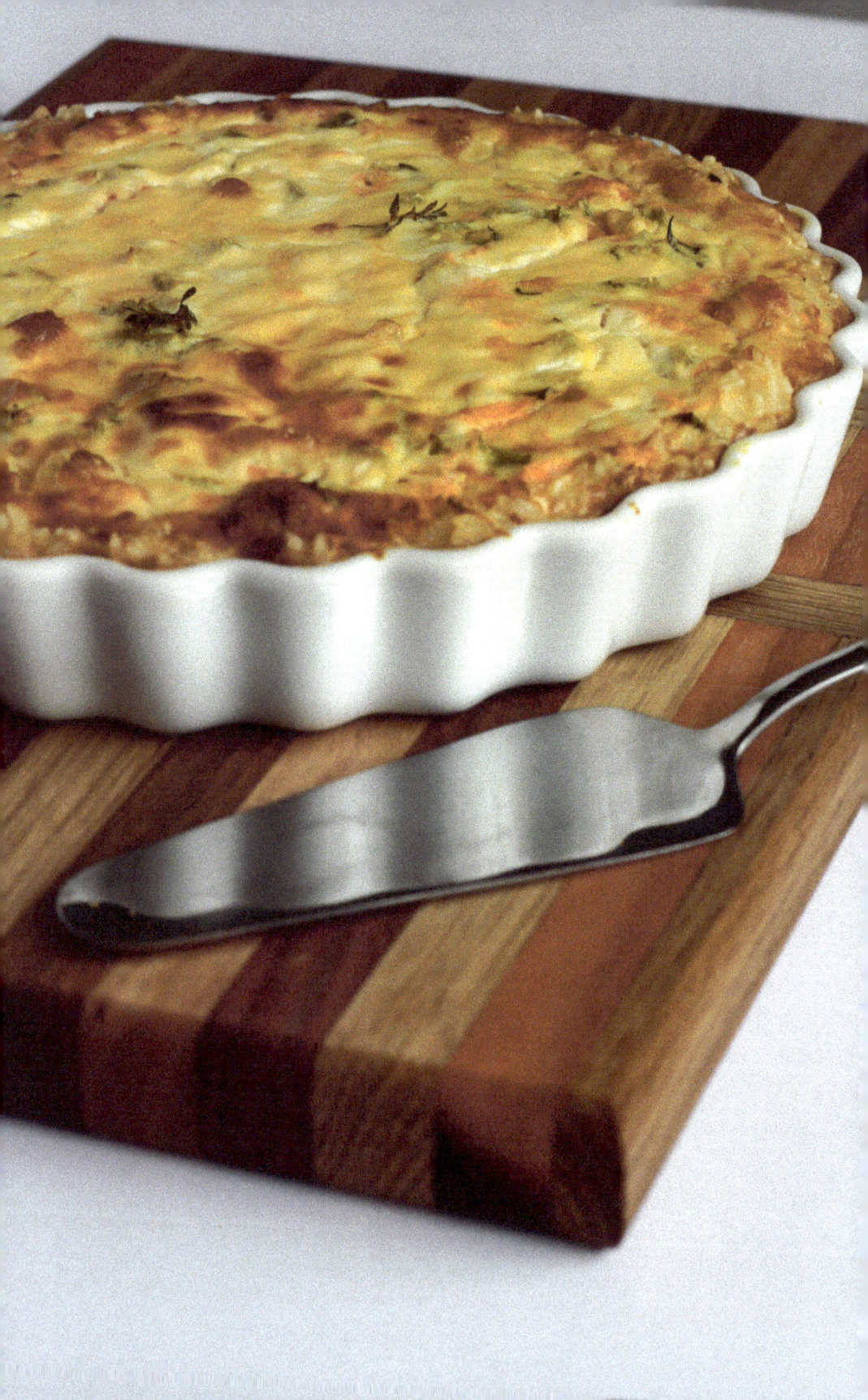

What foods have been avoided in this book?

None of the following ingredients are used in ANY recipe throughout this book:

gluten, wheat flour, oats, barley, rye

dairy products

peanuts and all other nuts

sesame seeds

shellfish

processed meats and sauces

yeast

vinegar

caffeine

additives, preservatives, colours, MSG

coconut

mushrooms

chocolate

refined sugar and artificial sweeteners

Why I Wrote This Book

My Food Intolerance Journey

My name is Cheree and I am not a chef, a business owner, a model, actress, celebrity, blogger or any other type of person you'd expect to write a cookbook. I am actually a 66-year-old wife, mother and grandmother. A regular, everyday person – just like you. I am someone who has always loved sewing, all types of craft, art work and my biggest passion: cooking and appreciating good food.

I also have coeliac disease, am lactose intolerant and have a number of other food intolerances which, unfortunately, were not diagnosed until I was 49 years of age.

From the age of four until 49, I had a constant battle with my health. I suffered with migraines, itchy sensitive skin, stomach pain, sinus pain, throat infections, travel sickness, bowel problems and bloating. As I got older, the symptoms got worse - especially the awful migraines. They would begin with white glowing spots in front of my eyes, then I would go numb on one side of my face and slur my words. When the headache came, the pain would be on the reverse side of the numbness and then the numbness would go. I would have to spend a day in a dark room and slowly the pain would subside. Finally, it would result in another couple of days feeling sore and sluggish. Everyone said I would grow out of it but unfortunately as I got older the migraines just become more frequent. This was no way to live.

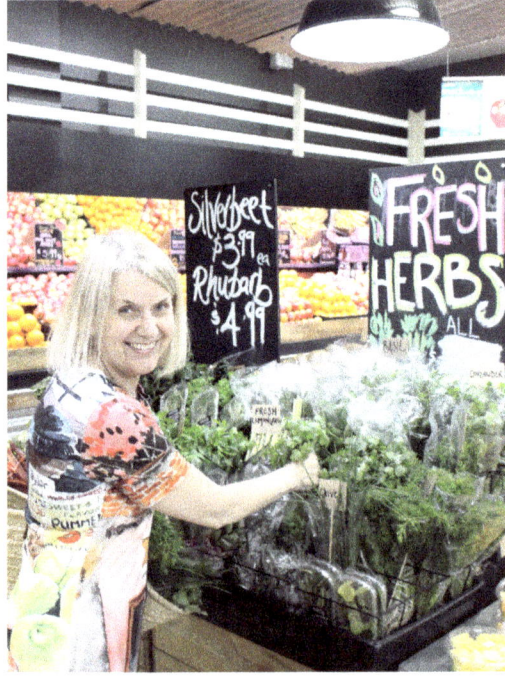

As a teenager I was told it was hormonal; in my twenties pregnancy was blamed; then stress as we moved often with my husband's work. When I reached my forties the symptoms must, of course, be menopause. I had been to doctors, neurologists and specialists of all kinds. I had CT scans, angiograms, and blood tests but nothing showed up to give a diagnosis. Everyone was very kind, but apart from antibiotics and migraine tablets no one was able to help me. By now, my migraines were coming fortnightly and the numbness was progressing. It was going down one side of my face and my body. All my other problems were also getting more severe.

My motto had always been 'this is your lot – just live with it, put up with it and work around it' but now my quality of life was being severely affected. I couldn't spend half my life in a dark room and going to doctors, I had a busy life and a life I wanted to enjoy. I was getting desperate.

A Solution

By chance, I saw an advertisement in our local paper about a nutritionist. It talked about food allergies and food intolerances and the symptoms that arise from them. It could have been written about me – the symptoms were all so familiar – so I made an appointment.

From that very first visit my entire life changed. I found all my health problems were caused by food and this meant they could be controlled by food. Not only did I need a gluten-free and lactose-free diet, but after years of being on antibiotics and being so ill, I also had candida (thrush) and my immune system was extremely low and needed building up.

The list of food that I couldn't eat seemed endless: wheat, oats, barley, rye, gluten, malt, dairy milk, cream, ice-cream, all types of cheeses, sugar (in any form whilst I had candida and also many types of fruit), artificial sweeteners, yeast, vinegar, caffeine, chocolate, takeaway food, processed meats and sauces, preservatives, colours, additives, MSG, peanuts, sesame seeds, mushrooms, coconut and high acid fruits (for my itchy skin) such as pineapple, strawberries, orange, mandarin, kiwi fruit, strawberries and apples.

I went back to my doctor to have my gluten intolerance confirmed and after tests it was official. I was coeliac. Unfortunately because my migraines had been the doctor's and specialist's main concern, and as coeliac disease was a relatively new health condition at the time, it had been overlooked.

Within just three weeks of cutting these foods from my diet I felt amazing - without gluten the migraines and bloating were gone, the itchy skin was getting better, my bowel was finally behaving normally and without milk and cheese in my diet my sinus, sore teeth and sore throat was gone.

Starting Over

Life was great BUT I so very much missed eating all the great meals I had once enjoyed – now all my meals were bland and very boring as all my favourite foods were off limits. Eating wasn't any fun and cooking, which had once been such a great passion, was now undertaken for the rest of the family to enjoy.
I thought the days of eating and cooking good food for myself were gone. It was so sad that I was cooking delicious food for everyone else and my meals were so terribly tasteless.

I looked for recipe books that might help my diet but alas, even though there were recipe books for Gluten-free OR Lactose/Dairy-free, there was nothing that combined the two and certainly there wasn't anything that also included recipes that were free from nuts, vinegar, refined sugar, yeast, acid fruits, coconut etc.

I then decided it was time to create my own recipes. I did it all the time for my family so why couldn't I make my CAN EAT food list into edible, enjoyable meals for

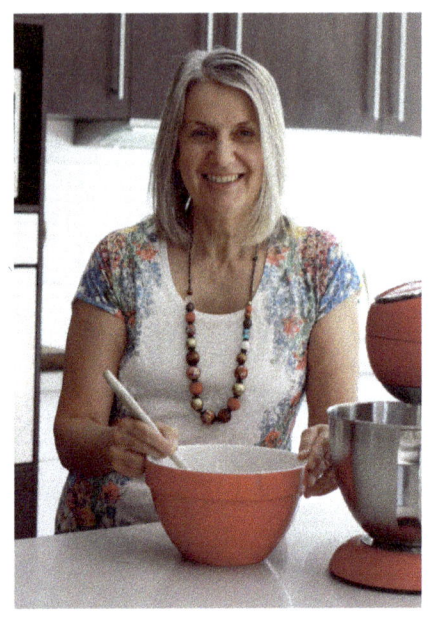

everyone? Who knows, they might eventually taste delicious and the whole family, my friends and other people with food problems could eat them (and not even know)!

The first step was discovering exactly what ingredients were in everything and what I could use in place of the foods that I needed to steer clear of. Once the list stared growing, ever so slowly, I started to experiment by changing my old favourites and substituting different ingredients for foods I could have. I had a lot of failures, and a lot of laughs but after a while I had a small collection of recipes.

I wanted to help other people like me so I decided to self-publish my own cookbook and sell it online.

With my daughter's help we created *Who Said I Can't Eat That* - a small cookbook that was sold in Australia, New Zealand, England, Ireland and America. I was amazed how well the book was received. It was great to get emails from people who had similar problems to mine and to hear that I had been able to help them.

This made me decide that I needed to understand more about allergies, diet and nutrition so I embarked on studying. I took two courses – Diet and Nutrition, and Food and Envirionmental Allergies. I found them both very interesting and challenging. I was delighted when I finally completed them and was presented with two diplomas.

Today

A lot has changed in the food world since my original diagnosis. Gluten-free pasta doesn't taste like chewy cardboard, dairy substitutes are abundant and the Paleo craze has ensured there are a lot of food options for people with restrictions (although many Paleo recipes do use a lot of coconut which isn't good for people with food intolerances). However, I have realised there is still a challenge for those of us with multiple food intolerances. It is still difficult for the person cooking for their family when one child is coeliac; another is allergic to dairy and a third has diabetes (yes, those unlucky types do exist!). I realised that my recipes are more important today than ever. Wouldn't it be wonderful to make a meal – entrée, main AND dessert – that any person could eat and enjoy without worrying about accommodating food allergies or food intolerances? Wouldn't it be great to have a staple list of easy, yummy and inexpensive dishes that everyone could cook and eat without concern?

So, welcome to my revised and updated book…happy cooking and, most certainly, happy eating!

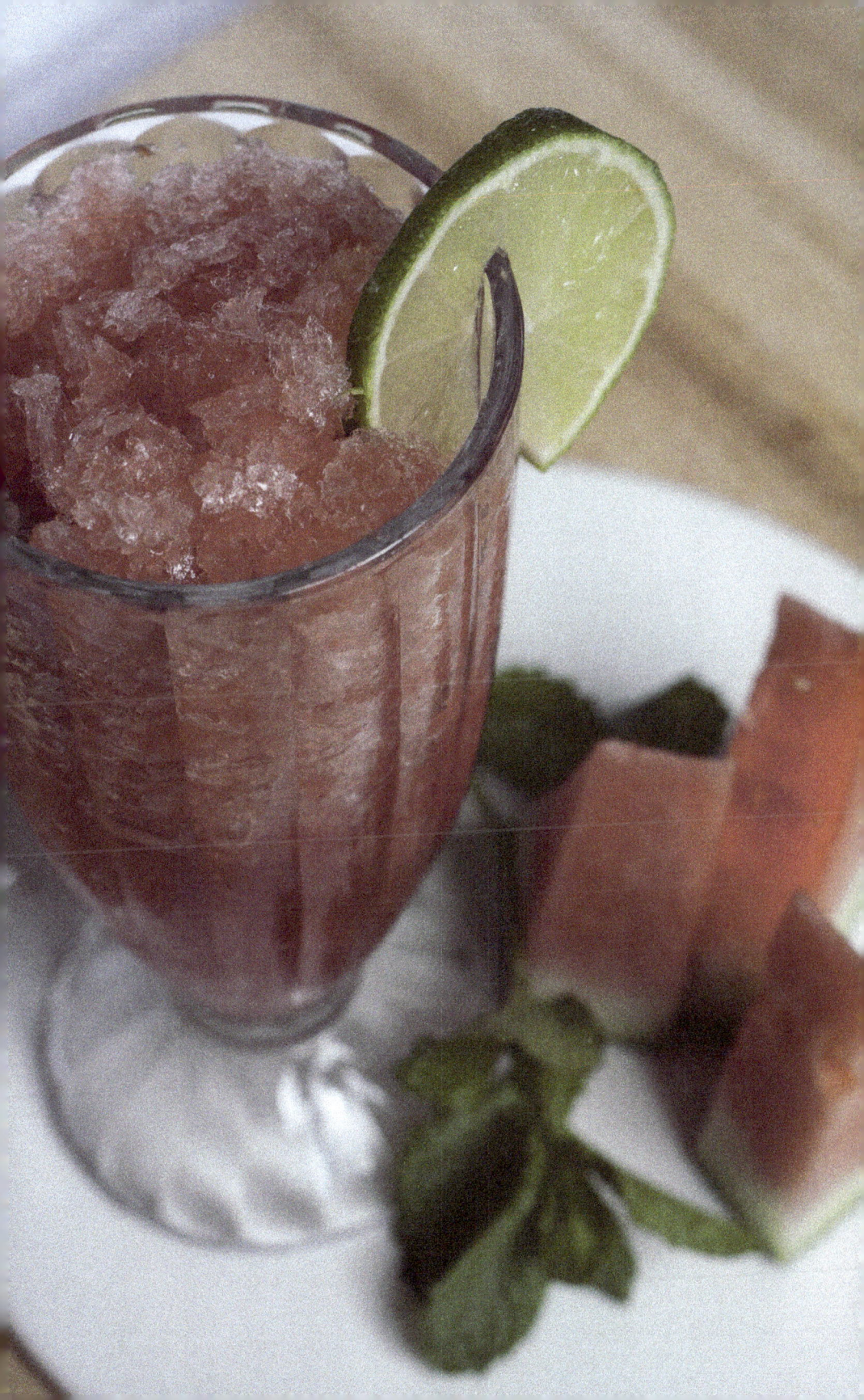

Finding Substitutes

Trying to recreate my favourite recipes using foods that I can eat has resulted in a great deal of trial and error! Hopefully, I can make life easier for you by sharing some of my secrets.

Flour

Instead of using wheat, oats, barley, rye or gluten I have used alternative wheat and flour products such as rice, maize, cornflour, soy, buckwheat, potato flour, gram flour and tapioca flour. Whilst these options can sometimes offer a similar texture or consistency as wheat flours, the taste will often vary and so will the results.

There are also fabulous gluten-free options at your supermarket these days, pre-mixed gluten-free self raising and plain flour work just as good as the non-gluten-free versions.

Dairy

When substituting dairy, I use soy milk (malt and sugar free), natural soy yoghurt (sometimes soy yoghurt without flavour is really hard to find!), vanilla soy yoghurt and blueberry soy yoghurt. Rice milk is great and it gives puddings, gelato, scones, etc a really nice texture and a sweet flavour (meaning less sugar, yay!) If you can tolerate dairy, I encourage you to continue to use butter, dairy milk, yoghurt, etc as it still remains one of the best sources of calcium.

Sugar

These days, many people will tell you that sugar is the enemy. It's become so excessive that a lot of people will say that you shouldn't even be eating fruit. My take is that everything is OK in moderation. The secret is to source the foods that have the least amount of processes taking place to achieve the final result! And really, if you already have a large list of foods that you 'can't' eat for fear of them making you sick, having someone tell you that fruit is bad too is enough to send you completely round the twist!

I have used fruit sugar or fructose, which is unrefined sugar from fruit; rice syrup and pure Canadian maple syrup. All of these are low GI (five times lower than refined sugar) and are therefore released more slowly into your system rather than an instant artificial sugar hit!

A diet high in sugar certainly has a negative effect on your skin and your immune system. Almost everything on the shelves in the supermarket contains sugar and it is addictive – the more you have, the more you want. When you eliminate processed sugar from your diet, everything starts to taste so much better. Your taste buds will become more sensitive to the natural sweetness in food and as your cravings dwindle, you will become calmer. Just remember that it's refined sugar you want to avoid. Be wary of new products on the market: Stevia is promoted as natural but it's highly processed and just as addictive as artificial sugar and agave

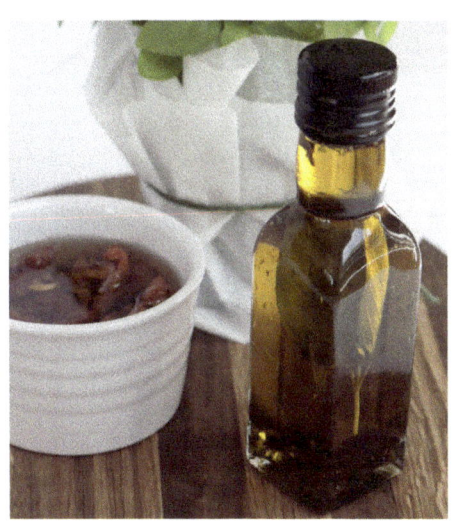

syrup has a very highest fructose content and therefore doesn't metabolise well. Like everything in life, just keep it simple and you'll be fine.

Cooking With Oils

When making starters, soups and mains I tend to use cold pressed, extra virgin olive oil. It's easy to find, nutritious and can be used both cold and heated. When I need an extra high temperature (for example, in a stir fry) I use rice bran oil instead, as olive oil tends to smoke.

When baking desserts, I like to use sunflower or safflower oil, or a vegan spread. Instead of vinegar, I use lime or lemon juice – they are a great source of phosphorus and help to repair the nervous system. They also have sodium to purify the liver and vitamins A and C that will protect from colds, aid circulation and brighten the eyes.

Meat

Many meats today are processed and I try to avoid them as much as possible. I used chemical-free meats and free-range, chemical-free poultry. Many butchers now will sell chemical-free meats as well as gluten-free options.

Additives & Preservatives

I use herbs and spices a lot – they enhance the flavour of your food and they have great health benefits for your body as well. Many premixed and premade sauces and seasonings have added preservatives or MSG which isn't ideal when you have immunity issues. A well stocked herb and spice rack makes life just as simple (and cheaper in the long run!) without the problems that come with all those additives. I go into a little more detail about herbs and spices over the page.

Extra Advice

Try to avoid caffeine if you can – stick to herbal teas that are caffeine free. Caffeine will irritate your immune system and make all those allergies and intolerances so much worse. Drink a lot of water – it will keep your body hydrated and your skin moist.

Eat seasonal fruit and vegetables - they will have been grown closer to home and therefore are less likely to have been treated with a lot of chemicals for longevity. Fruit and vege in season is also a lot less expensive!

Where possible, go for home-grown or organic options so that you know what you are eating is chemical free.

Don't be afraid to have a go at altering your favourite recipe to suit your diet! You might be surprised at what you are able to create…and how easy it actually is.

How To Add Flavour

When you're not using any additives, preservatives or colours in recipes, you have to rely on natural herbs and spices for taste and colour.

With the growing concern of side effects from chemical colours, additives and preservatives in our food today, I can promise that delicious herbs and spices can transform an ordinary dish into a culinary delight. It also provides a natural, healthy and nutritious way of cooking. Herbs can be used fresh or dried (although I would recommend growing your own herbs either in pots or as a herb garden in the yard). Having fresh herbs handy helps with cooking and it is a rewarding, aromatic and pleasurable experience. If space or time restricts you, you can always buy fresh or dried herbs from supermarkets or health shops. Dried herbs are fine and will certainly help you add the flavour you need but, just like the difference in taste between fruit and vegetables from the supermarket compared to those straight from the tree, you will really notice a difference with fresh herbs.

HERBS

Herbs are the leaves of small plants (as opposed to a spice which is a dried root, seed, fruit, vegetable or bark) used to give additional flavour to food. They're also great for herbal teas, herbal baths and have many other uses - but that would be another book - so for now I will give you a guide through the herbs (and spices) that I use most when cooking.

Anise/Aniseed

The seeds give a pleasant liquorice taste to many types of foods. Use whole or crushed in breads, cakes, apple pies, apple sauce, creams and confectionary. Add to pickles, curries and water when boiling shellfish. Chew slightly roasted seed after a meal as a breath sweetener or as a good tonic for the digestive system. The flower can be mixed into fruit salads. The leaf can be used as a garnish. The stem and root can be mixed into soups and stews for a hint of liquorice.

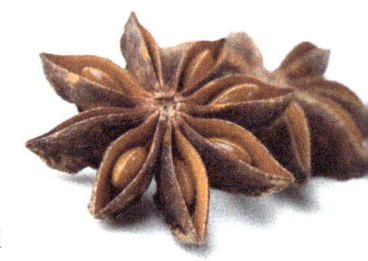

Bay Leaf

The leaf of the Sweet Bay Tree can be used fresh or dried. Excellent as flavouring in soups, stews, sauces and custards (just remember to remove the leaf before eating). Bay leaves are an essential component of the "bouquet garni" (see end of section – page 17). This can be used as a garnish, or kept in your rice storage jar to flavour rice.

It's also an old belief that no harm can come to a house where a bay tree grows.

Basil

Basil is my favourite herb. It's warm spicy flavour and pungent aroma is sensational and you will notice in my recipes that I use it a lot. Add leaves to soups, sauces and tomato and garlic dishes. Basil tea is a useful remedy for travel sickness. It's also a natural mosquito repellent (just rub fresh leaves into the skin).

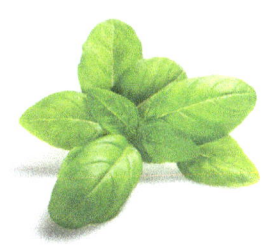

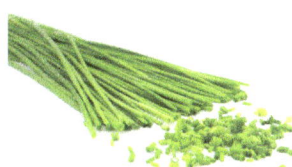

Chervil

Chervil has a delicate parsley type flavour. Use generously in salads, soups, sauces, vegetable, chicken, white fish and egg dishes. Add chervil freshly chopped near the end of cooking to avoid flavour loss, or use it to garnish foods.

Coriander

The dried seed is used in tomato chutney, ratatouille and curries. The fresh lower leaves can be added to oriental and curry dishes, stews, salads, sauces and used as a garnish.

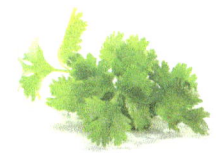

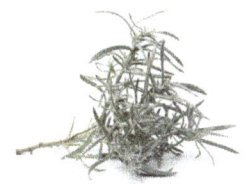

Chives

A very small type of onion, the green leaves of chives have a delicate onion flavour. The leaves are chopped to flavour eggs, potatoes, soups, salads, sauces, butter and cheeses. Add the fresh flowers to salads.
To reconstitute dried chives moisten with salad dressing or lemon juice.

Curry plant

This is a relatively new addition to the herbal list. Add a leaf sprig to soups, stews, steamed vegetables, rice dishes and pickles for a mild curry flavour. Remove sprig before serving.

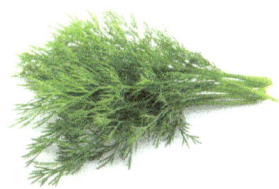

Dill

Use the seed of dill whole or ground in soups, fish dishes, pickles, cabbage, apple pies, dill butter, cakes and breads. Add the young, green seed heads to potato salad. Use the finely chopped leaf to flavour soups, salads, eggs, salmon and grilled meats or use as a garnish. Boil with new potatoes.

Fennel

Fennel seed is used in sauces, fish dishes and bread. The leaf (finely chopped) is used over salad and cooked vegetables. It's also a nice addition to soups.

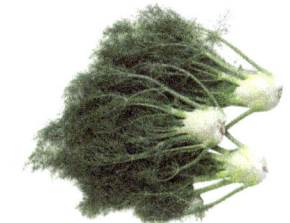

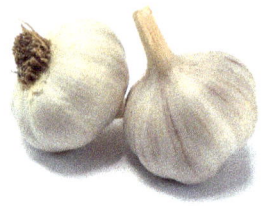

Garlic
Garlic is one of the most useful herbs in the kitchen and home grown tastes terrific. Use the bulb (cloves) with meat, soup, vegetables and savoury dishes. The leaves and flowers have a milder garlic taste, add them to salads and stir fries. When eaten, garlic can fight infection and reduce blood pressure.

Lavender (English)
Remove the flowers and add to jams, sweet dishes, cream and biscuits. There are other varieties of lavender but the English Lavender is the only one you can use in your cooking.

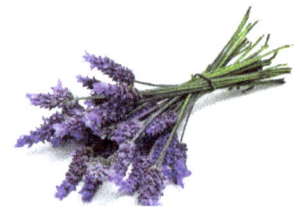

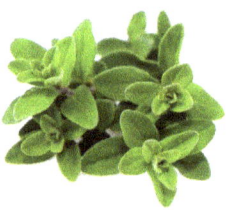

Mint
The green leaves of the spearmint plant have a fresh scent. Sprigs are used when cooking new potatoes and peas. Chopped mint may be served in salads, and for mint sauce served with roast lamb. It adds a refreshing flavour to various fruit drinks and fruit salads.

Marjoram
With its sweet and mild flavour, marjoram is one of the most compatible herbs. Sweet marjoram leaves are chopped finely for salads and butters. Add to meat dishes in last few minutes. Use in Bouquet Garni.

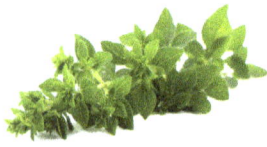

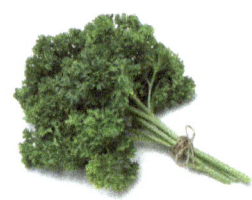

Oregano
With quite a pungent flavour it is used in many Mediterranean dishes, particularly pizza toppings and pasta sauces. Compliments basil in lasagne and tomato dishes.

Parsley
The most usual types are curly leaf and flat leaf (Italian 'continental' and French parsley). Fresh tasting and aromatic, parsley flavours most dishes. Chew raw to freshen breath and promote healthy skin. Also great as a garnish. Use in Bouquet Garni.

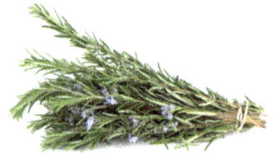

Rosemary
With its fresh pine fragrance, you can toss flowers into salads. Add leaf sparingly to a wide range of meat, especially lamb and pork. Great with baked potatoes, herbed butter, herbed bread and scones.

Sage
Scatter the flower in salads. The leaf is good in poultry stuffing or added to hot oil or butter to make a delicious sauce or dip.

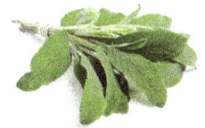

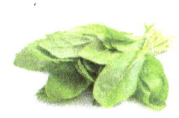

Sorrel
When cooked and pureed, it can be added to sauces for fish or poultry, and to potatoes or soup.

Tarragon
Shred the leaf and add to avocado fillings, mayonnaise, salad dressings, light soups, tomatoes, omelettes, scrambled eggs. Use to make herb butter.

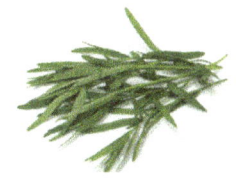

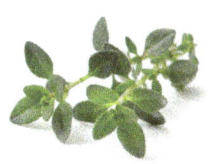

Thyme
Use young leaves to make stocks, marinades, stuffing, stews, sauces and soups. Use sparingly as it has a strong flavour. Attracts butterflies to your garden. Use in Bouquet Garni.

Bouquet Garni or Cook's Bunch
This is a bunch of mixed herbs tied together with white cotton or string and placed in a muslin bag. Add to soups and casseroles for a wonderful flavour.
Consists of 3 sprigs of parsley, 2 sprigs of thyme, 1 sprig marjoram, 1 bay leaf.

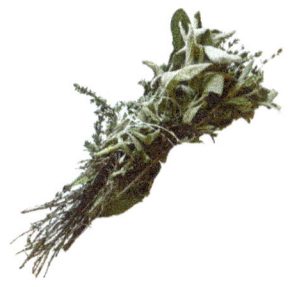

SPICES

All Spice
This is the berry of evergreen pimento tree grown in the West Indies and South America, and combines the flavours of cloves, nutmeg and cinnamon. The berries are used whole or ground as a flavouring for pickles, sauces, meat dishes, stock and fruit puddings.

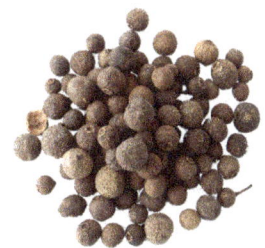

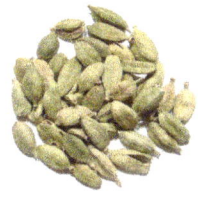

Cardamom
Grown in the tropics, seeds are used to flavour marinade, punches, etc. Ground seeds are good for fruit salads, curries cakes, breads and biscuits.

Cinnamon

A spice obtained from the inner bark of several trees from the genus Cinnamomum that is used in both sweet and savoury foods. It is used in stick form or as a powder to flavour sweet dishes and cakes.

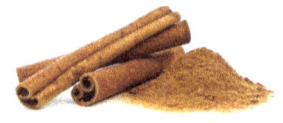

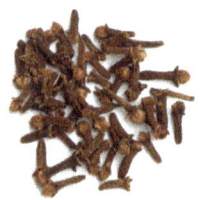

Cloves

The dried unopened flower buds of an evergreen tree grown in tropical climates. Whole cloves are used to flavour apples, pears, chutney and savoury dishes. Ground cloves are used in some cakes and biscuits.

Cumin

Mostly produced in India, these are powerful flavoured seeds (whole or ground) and added to many Middle Eastern and Indian dishes like lamb, curries and yoghurt.

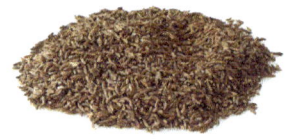

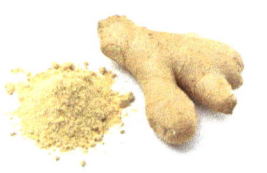

Ginger

This is a root grown in Brazil and West Indies. It can be preserved or dried in a powdered form as ground ginger. Fresh ginger root peeled, sliced or grated can be added to stews, sauces and oriental dishes. Use ground ginger in cakes, biscuits and puddings.

Nutmeg

The kernel or the fruit of a tall evergreen tropical tree. Used grated for many sweet and savoury dishes or powdered for flavouring cakes, biscuits, puddings and milk dishes.

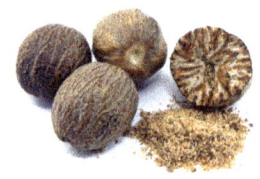

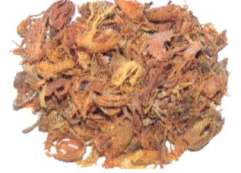

Mace

This is the outer covering of nutmeg, flattened and dried. It is used whole or in ground form to flavour fish, stock, sauces, stews and pickles.

Peppercorns

The dried berries of a plant grown in hot countries. Unground pepper berries keep their flavour better than ground pepper. Used for stews, soups and pickles. A small pepper mill may be used for grinding peppercorns.

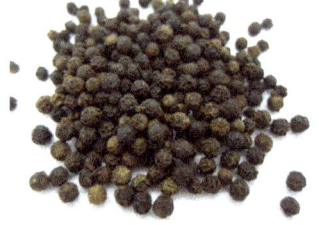

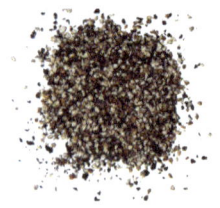

Black pepper

Black Pepper is made from the whole berry ground (white pepper is made from grinding the berries after the husks have been removed). Black pepper has a stronger flavour but gives a speckled appearance to food so white pepper is sometimes preferred as a condiment.

Cayenne Pepper

A hot bright red variety of pepper made from ground dried seeds and pods of chillies. The pepper takes its name from a town in South America where it originated. It is used discretely in highly seasoned dishes.

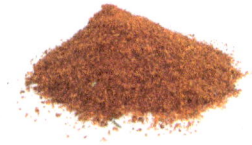

Paprika

A red pepper less strong than cayenne made from the Hungarian paprika. Used for flavouring and garnishing.

Saffron

Yellow in colour, this most delicately flavoured spice used to flavour and colour rice, meat and fish dishes, soup, bread, biscuits and cakes.

Vanilla

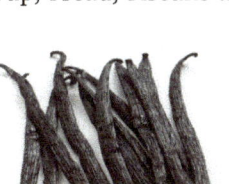

This is the dried fruit or pod of a type of orchid that grows in the tropics. Dried, cured fruit pods known as vanilla pods are used in custards and sweets. Vanilla extract is made by soaking the pods in alcohol.

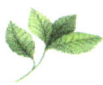

Freezing Herbs

One of the best ways to 'store' fresh herbs is to freeze them. Freezing retains colour and flavour as well as most of the nutritional value of fresh young leaves. This is convenient and fast and also a more satisfactory method of preserving the more delicate culinary herb leaves such as fennel, chervil, parsley, basil*, tarragon and chives

The easiest way to freeze herbs is simply to pack them into plastic bags and label, either individually or in mixtures such as bouquet garni.

Store small packets in larger rigid containers in the freezer to avoid the possibility of them being lost or damaged.

Alternatively put finely chopped leaves into ice cube trays and top with water. One average cube holds 1 tablespoon (15ml or ½ fluid oz) of water - a convenient quantity for cooking. If the water is not required in a recipe, the ice cube can be placed in a sieve over a bowl and allowed to thaw.

* When freezing basil you need to paint the leaves both sides with olive oil to retain flavour.

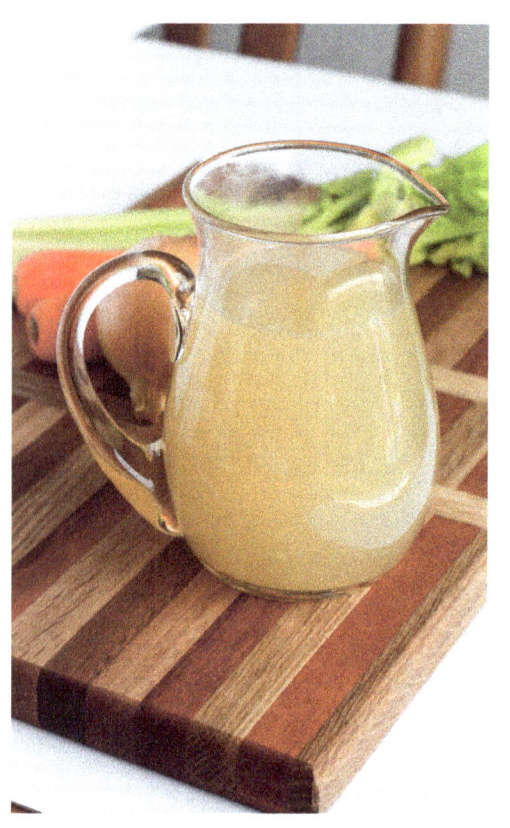
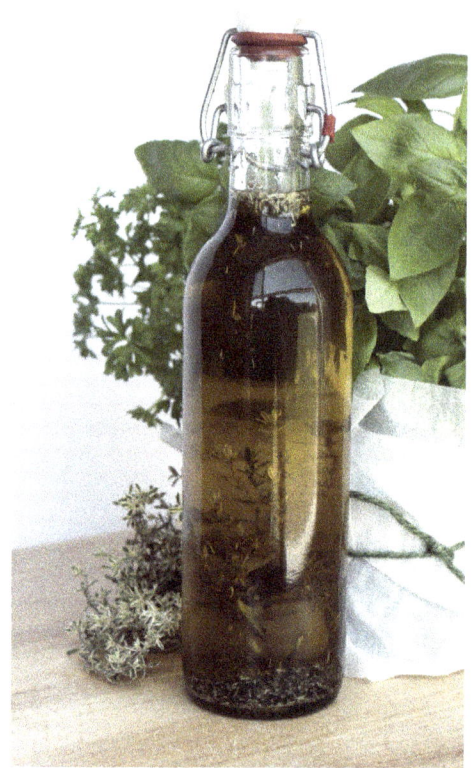
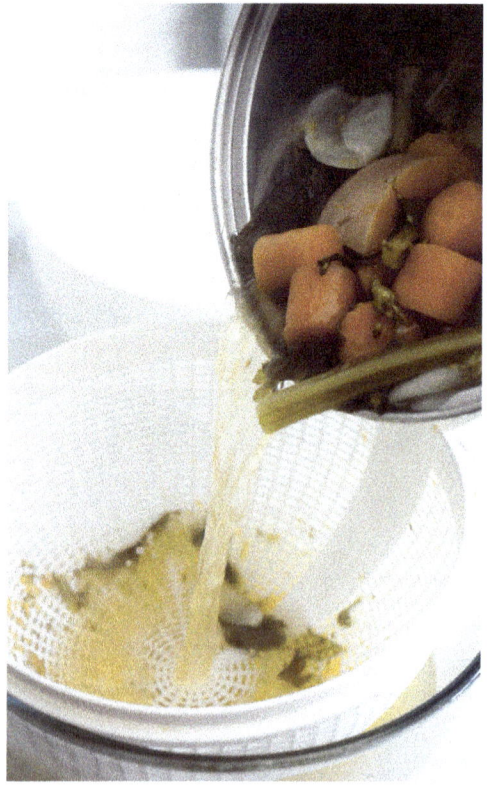
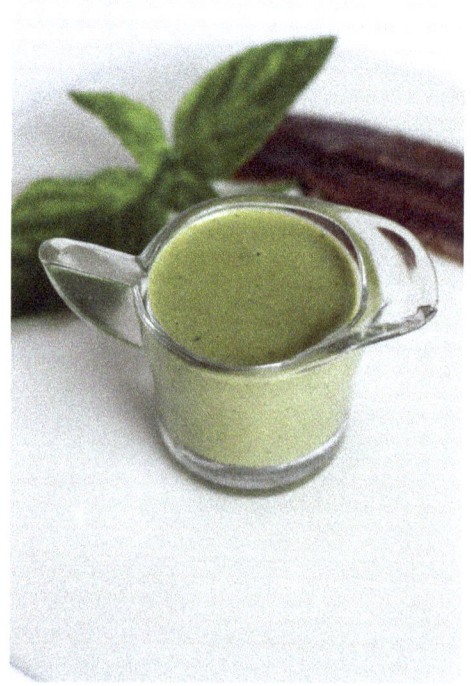

EXTRAS

These recipes really create the key ingredients for many of the dishes throughout this book - oils, sauces and stocks that are great to have in the fridge or freezer and can be used at any time to add flavour or make the perfect base for your meal.

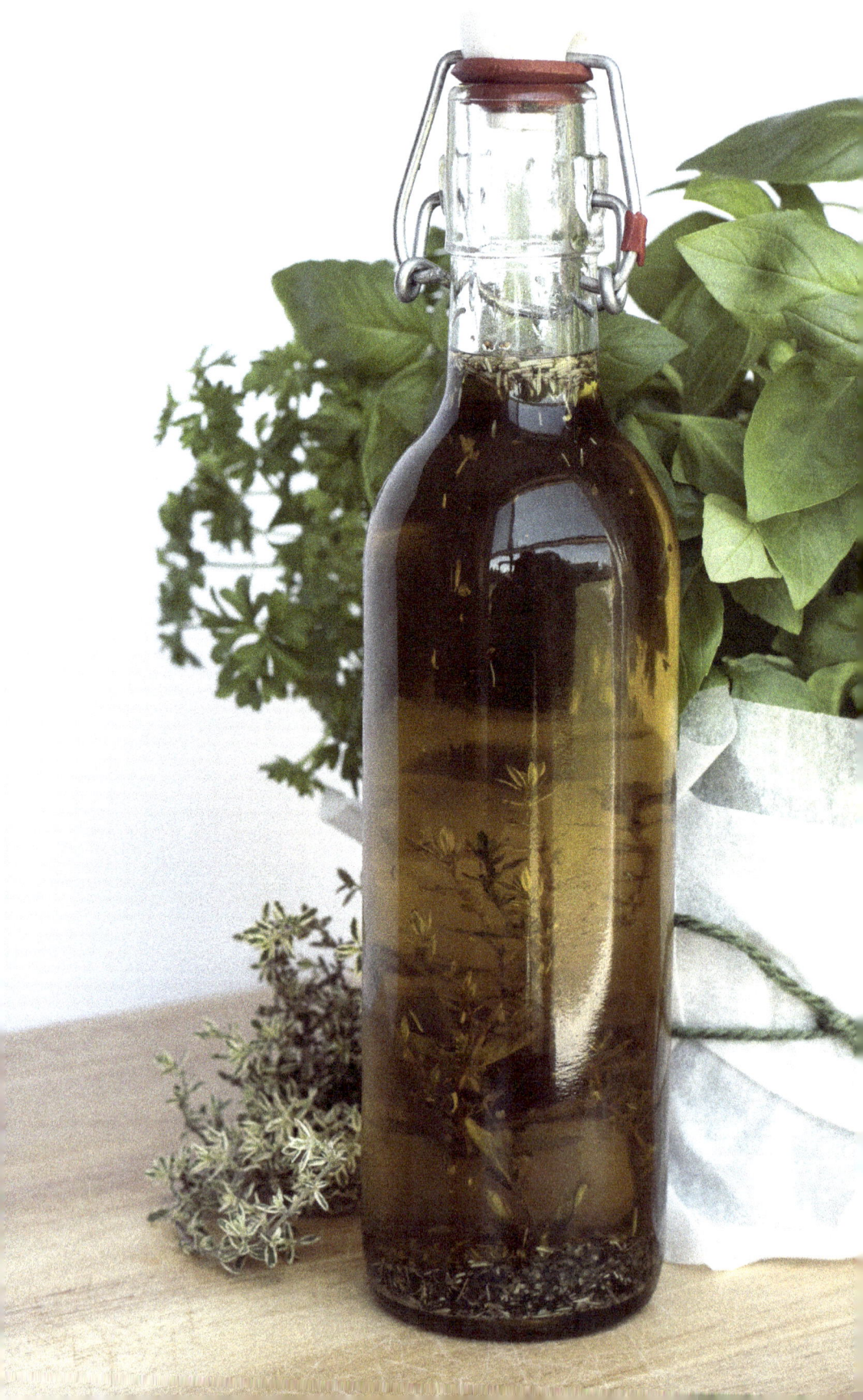

Herbed Oil

This is great for drizzling over a dish of pasta, for dipping breads into, for salads, for marinades, for cooking stir fries and sautéing. It is also very quick and easy to make.

INGREDIENTS
- Several large sprigs of fresh herbs (for example use rosemary, thyme, oregano, tarragon or sage (saving one or two sprigs to add later). Make sure they are washed and completely dry
- 2 cups olive oil

METHOD
1. Wash the herbs and pat dry. Leave them on a paper towel in the sun until completely dry or spread them out on a tray and heat them in the oven on low heat for a few minutes.
2. Push the herbs down into a clean dry, sterilised bottle, so the tips face upwards - don't cram in too many.
3. Fill the bottle up to the neck with oil and cover with a lid or cork.
4. Store in a cool place for 1 week.
5. Strain the oil into a jug through a muslin cloth or cheesecloth.
6. Pour the strained oil into a clean dry sterilised bottle, which has a couple of fresh dry herbs in it.
7. Store in the refrigerator for up to one week.
8. Once opened remove the large sprigs from the bottle as mould may grow on the herbs once they are not fully covered by the oil.
9. When ready to use take out of the refrigerator and allow the oil to come to room temperature.

NB. You can use dry or fresh herbs for this oil, but if using fresh herbs you need to make sure your herbs they are completely dry after washing, to prevent the herbs growing bacteria in them. Leave them in the sun for several hours or spread them on a tray and heat them in the oven on a low heat for a few minutes. Bacteria can't grow in the olive oil itself, but it can grow in the water left on the ingredients going into the oil.
Sterilise the jars or bottles by putting them through the dishwasher and then placing them in the oven on a low heat to dry them.

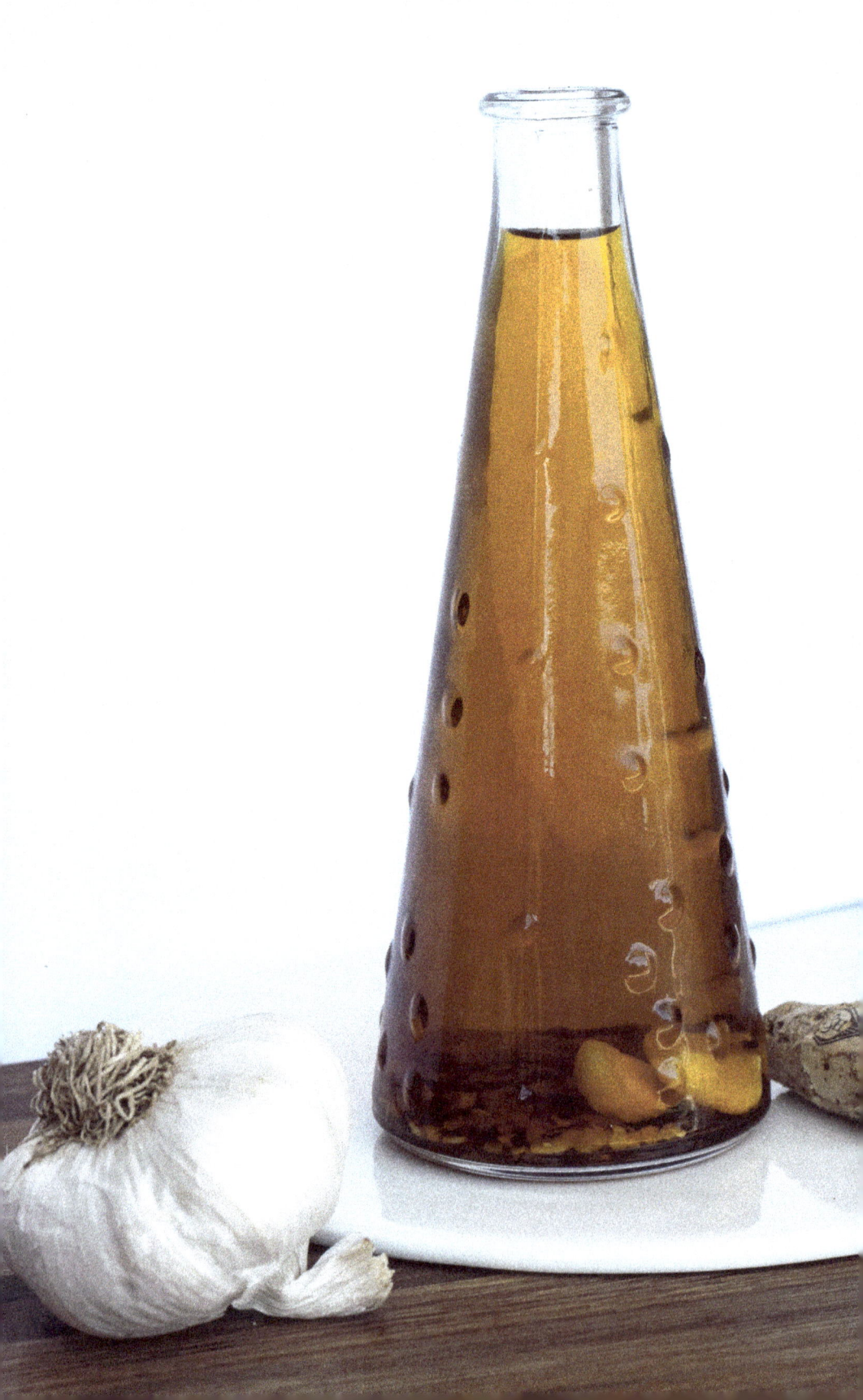

Garlic Infused Oil

I once used garlic butter with everything when I was cooking - it adds such great, great flavour. This oil is a wonderful alternative and, surprisingly, it's just as tasty and easy to work with. You don't have to use the chilli either…it's just as lovely without it but I like the extra kick!

INGREDIENTS
- 2 cups of olive oil
- 8 cloves of garlic smashed
- ¼ cup dried chilli flakes

METHOD
1. Pour enough of the olive oil in the bottom of your pan to cover the garlic gloves, add the garlic cloves and sauté over medium heat for 3-5 minutes. The garlic should sizzle but be careful not to burn it.
2. Add the rest of the olive oil and chilli flakes to the pan, bring down the heat to medium and simmer for 4 minutes.
3. Turn the heat down to low and simmer for 15 minutes.
4. Turn the heat off and let the oil cool down. Strain the oil into a jug through fine muslin cloth or cheesecloth and pour into a dry, sterilised bottle. Seal with a lid or cork and store in the refrigerator for 1 week.
5. Extra dried chilli flakes and dried crushed garlic can be inserted into the bottle before pouring in the strained oil if liked.
6. When ready to use allow the infused oil to come to room temperature.

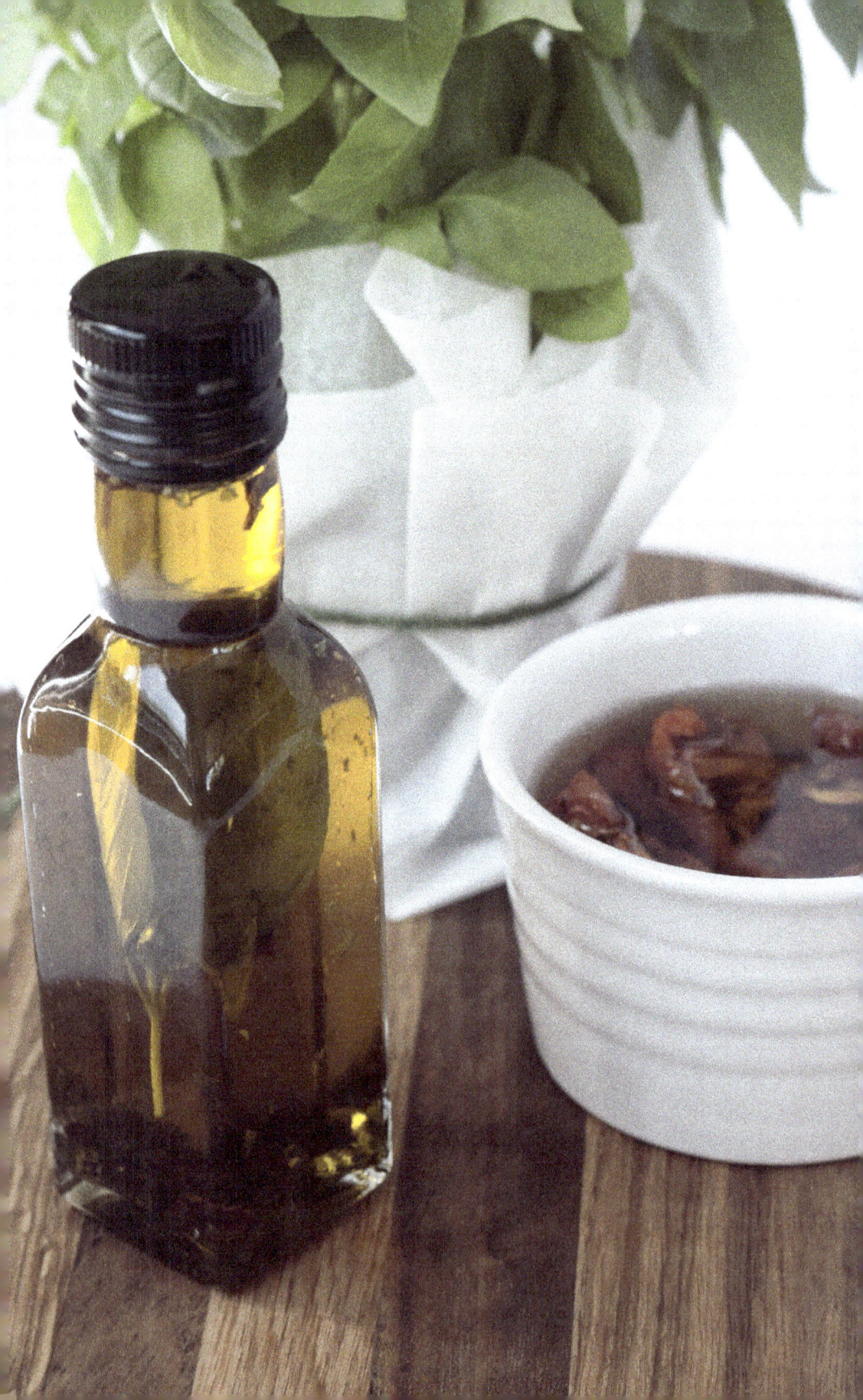

Basil & Tomato Oil

Basil is my favourite herb. With its sweet flavour, it is perfect for marinades or on a salad. I also love this oil over meat as a sauce.

INGREDIENTS
- 1 cup olive oil
- 1 ½ cups lightly packed fresh basil leaves
- 1 tablespoon finely chopped sun dried tomato

METHOD
1. Rinse and drain the basil leaves.
2. Pat the basil leaves dry with paper towel.
3. In a blender or food processor, combine the basil leaves and olive oil and whirl until the leaves are finely chopped (not pureed).
4. Pour the mixture into a saucepan and cook over medium heat, stirring occasionally until the oil bubbles around the sides of the pan (approximately 3-4 minutes).
5. Remove from the heat and let stand until cool (around 1 hour).
6. Line a fine wire strainer with two layers of fine muslin or cheesecloth and set over a small bowl.
7. Pour the oil mixture into the strainer.
8. After the oil is through, gently press the basil remaining in the cloth to release the remaining oil.
9. Discard the basil
10. Add the finely chopped sun dried tomato into the bottom of a dry sterilised jar or bottle. Pour the basil oil into the jar or bottle over the top of the sun dried tomato and cap or cork.
11. Store in the refrigerator for 1 week.
12. Bring the oil to room temperature before using.

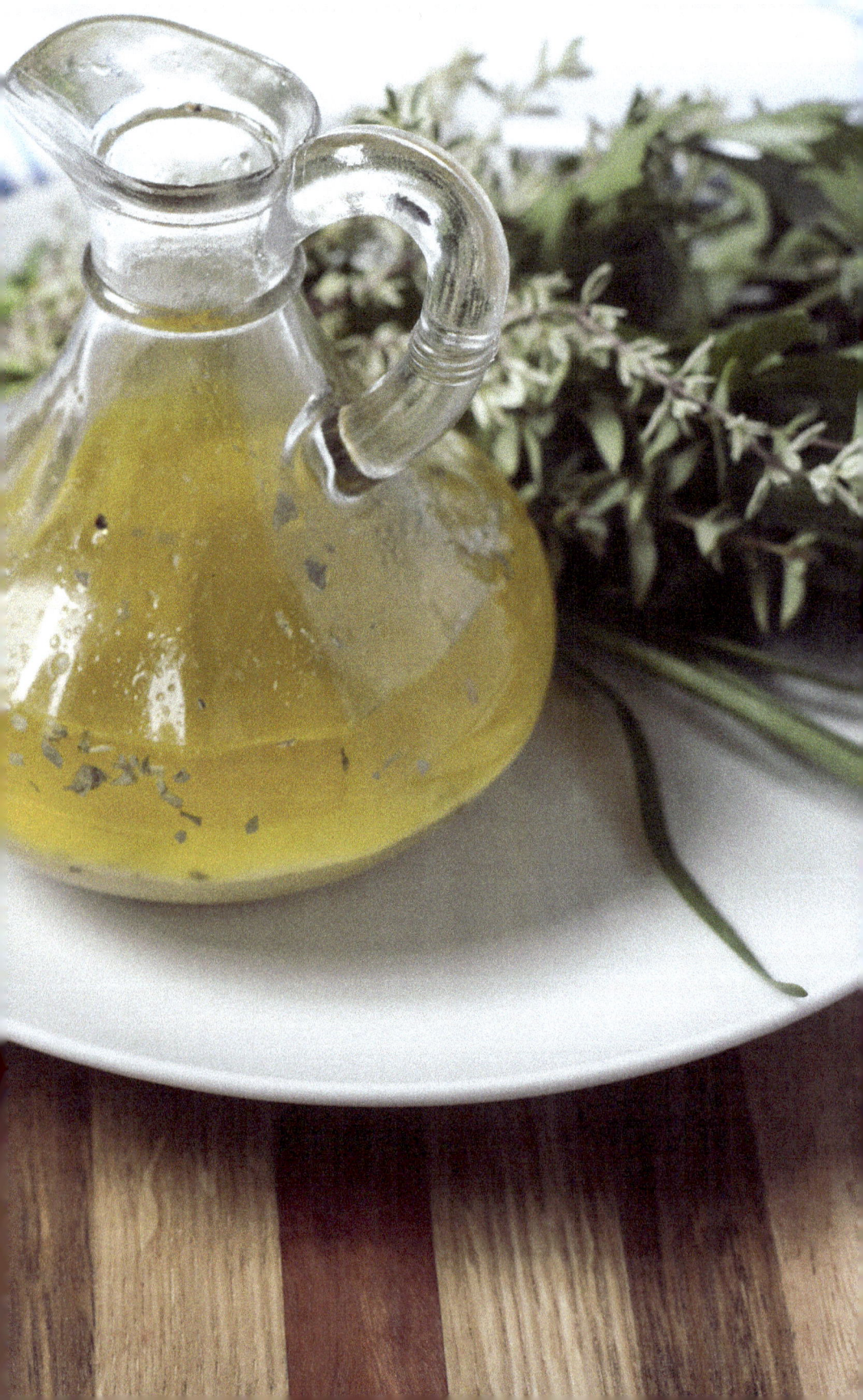

French Dressing

This simple dressing is all you need to make a salad pop. It gives a beautiful flavour if added to salad and main meat dish. It can also be used as a simple marinade for meats.

INGREDIENTS
- ¼ cup olive oil
- 2 tablespoons lemon or lime juice
- 1 crushed clove garlic
- ½ teaspoon sea salt
- ¼ teaspoon ground black pepper
- A pinch of dried chives, parsley, tarragon and thyme

METHOD
1. Soak crushed garlic in lemon or lime juice for ten minutes, strain lemon juice into a jar.
2. Place the rest of the ingredients in the jar, cover with a lid and shake well.
3. Store in the refrigerator for 1 week.

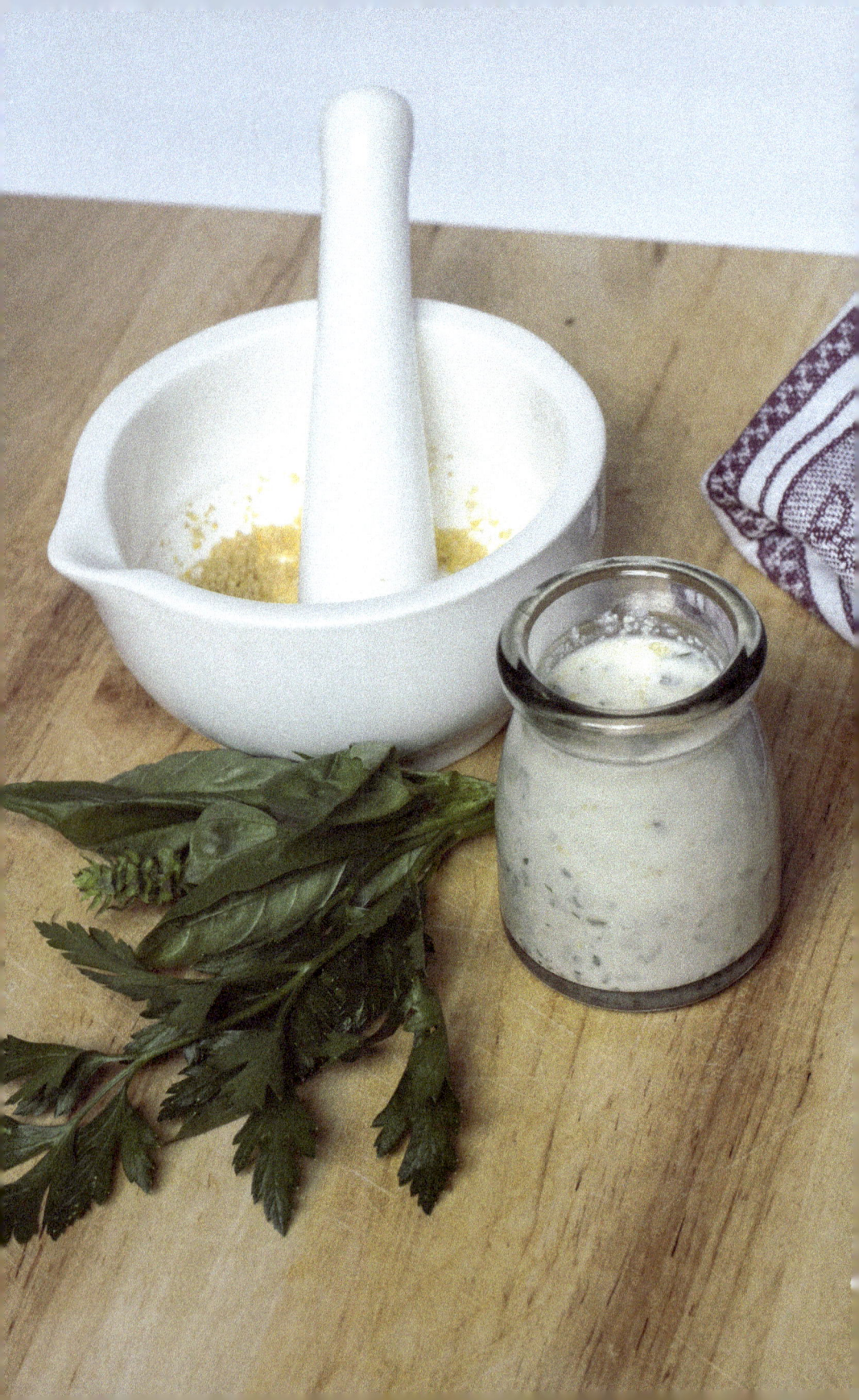

Mustard Sauce

Before I was sick, I always used a sauce to accompany my mains. Store-bought sauces are often not gluten-free and most mustard sauces have vinegar - another ingredient that was a no-no for me as it feeds candida - so I was determined to make my own. This sauce adds a lovely flavour to any meat or vegetable meal.

INGREDIENTS
- 3 teaspoons ground mustard seeds
- ¼ cup of chicken stock (see page 35)
- ¼ cup of natural soy yoghurt (or yoghurt of your choice)
- Freshly ground pepper for taste
- 1 tablespoon fresh finely chopped basil
- 1 tablespoon fresh finely chopped parsley

METHOD
1. Mix mustard seeds with the chicken stock.
2. Add all the other ingredients.
3. Mix well.
4. Store in a covered container in the refrigerator for 1 week.

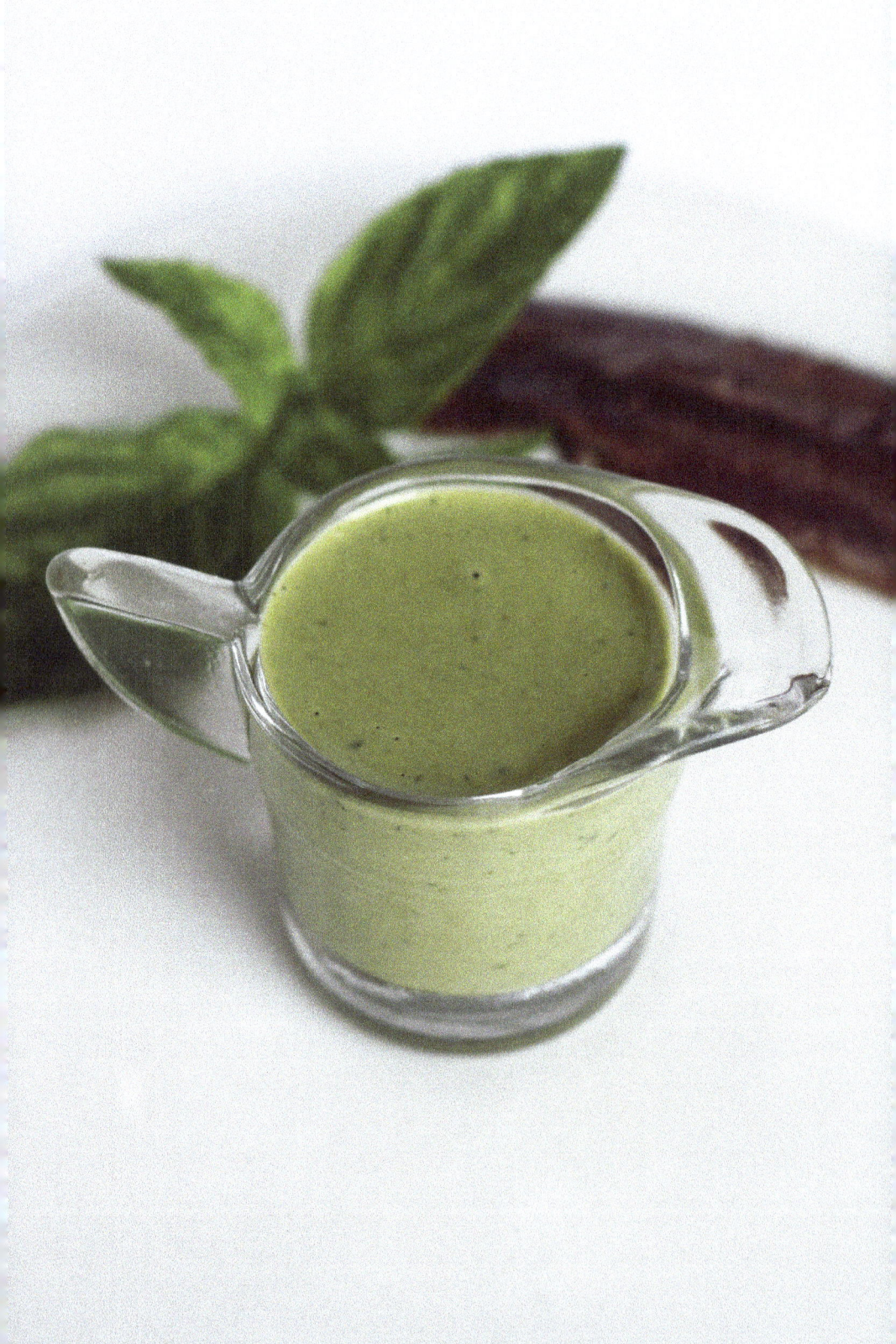

Anchovy Sauce

Don't be put off by the fact that anchovies are the key ingredients here - you know they are in Caesar salad dressing too? What it gives you is a lovely salty and creamy mix that tastes delicious with the freshness of the citrus and the combination of the garlic and herbs. It also adds the perfect zing to fish dishes.

INGREDIENTS
- 4 finely chopped anchovy fillets
- 1 clove garlic, peeled and crushed
- Zest and juice of 1 lemon or lime
- 3 tablespoons extra virgin olive oil
- 1 tablespoon fresh finely chopped parsley
- 1 tablespoon fresh finely chopped basil

METHOD
1. Put all ingredients in a food processor and blend until smooth and creamy.
2. Store in a covered container in refrigerator for 1 week.

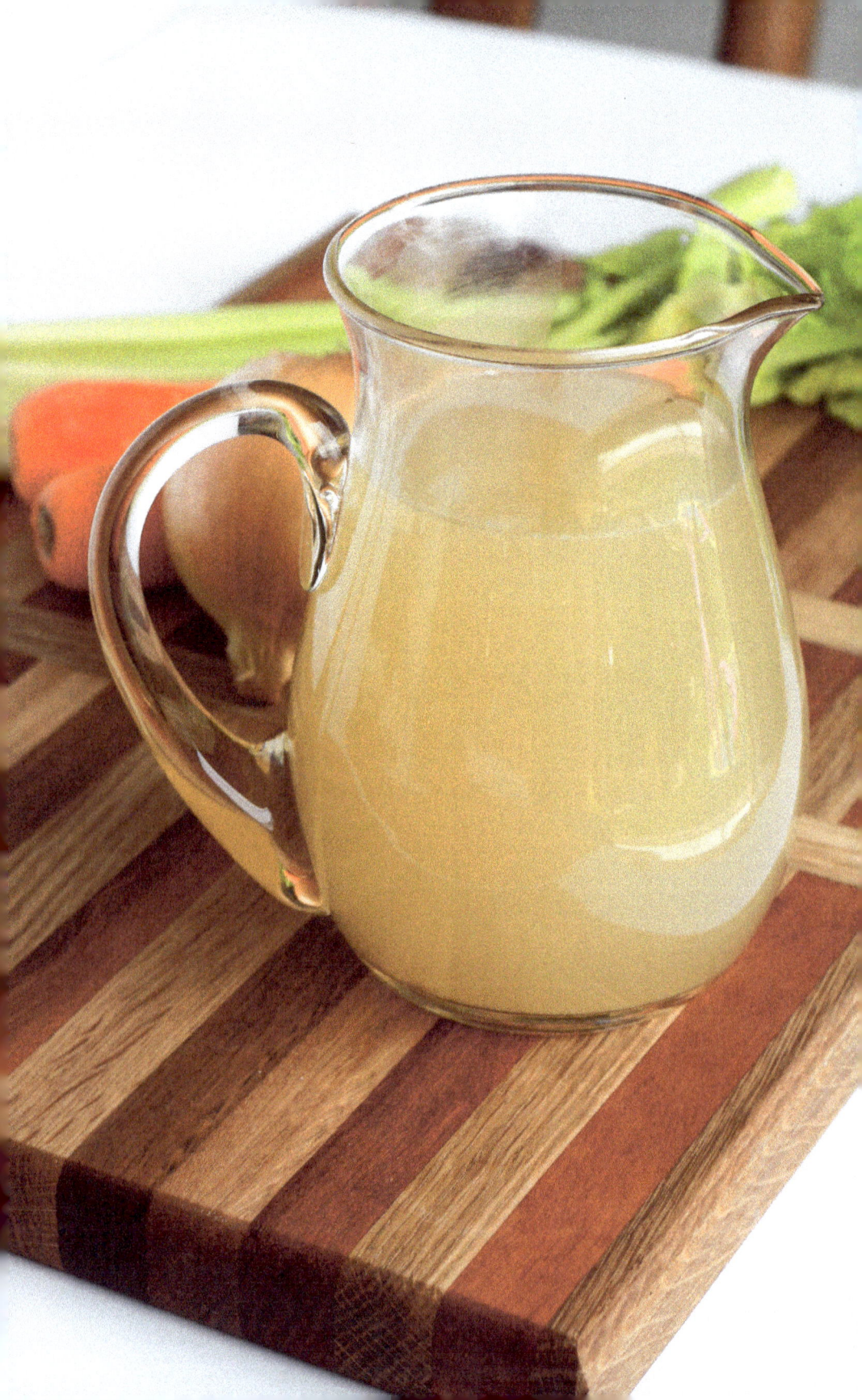

Chicken Stock

I would consider this an essential ingredient and you should always try to have some in your freezer ready to go. Whenever I make a batch, I measure and store the stock by the cup. I then freeze each cup individually and that makes it easy to throw a cup or two into any recipe that may need it.

INGREDIENTS
- 3 free range raw chicken carcasses
- 3 litres (6½ pints) of water
- 1 large onion, peeled and roughly chopped
- 2 garlic cloves peeled and chopped
- 2 stalks celery, chopped roughly
- 1 tablespoon fresh parsley, scissor chopped
- 1 tablespoon, fresh thyme, chopped
- 1 tablespoon fresh marjoram, scissor chopped
- 3 fresh bay leaves (or 2 dried)
- 12 whole black peppercorns

METHOD
1. Put all ingredients in a large pot and bring to the boil (these quantities will make approximately 14 cups).
2. Let simmer for 3 to 3½ hours. (If chicken carcasses are precooked simmer for 1 to 1½ hours)
3. Strain and place in refrigerator.
4. When cool, remove excess fat.
5. Put into containers and freeze until required (up to 3 months).

Tip: mark how many cups are in each container for easy defrosting to suit your planned meal.

*If stored in the refrigerator use within 2 days.

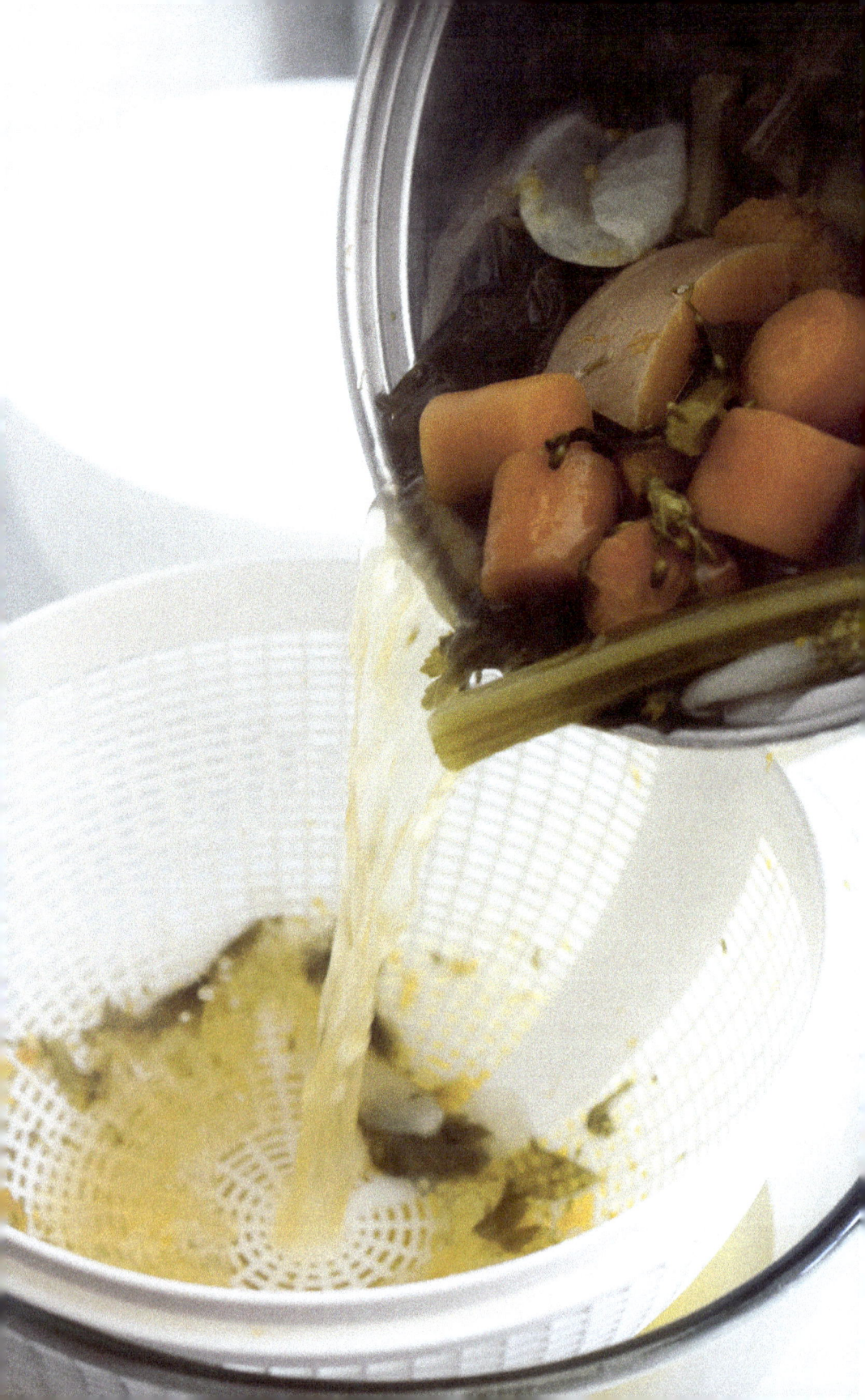

Vegetable Stock

This is a great way to use up leftover vegetables (it doesn't matter how sad they are looking, just throw them in!) and with no meat this will keep for ages in the fridge (around five days) and the freezer (approximately six months).

INGREDIENTS
- 2 litres water
- Head of a bunch of celery
- 2 onions peeled and chopped
- 1 large carrot, chopped
- 1 large parsnip, chopped
- 1 cup beans, chopped
- 2 potatoes, chopped
- 2 cups pumpkin
- 1 bouquet garni
- 1 teaspoon sea salt
- 6 whole black peppercorns
- 2 bay leaves

METHOD
1. Combine all ingredients in a large pot, bring to the boil, then simmer for 45 minutes.
2. Strain into a non metallic container and cool
3. When the stock is cold cover and store in the refrigerator for up to 4 days , or freeze for later use.
4. Keep in the freezer for 6 months.

* The vegetables and herbs I have used are just a guide, you can use any vegetables you have on hand so experiment and see what you can come up with!

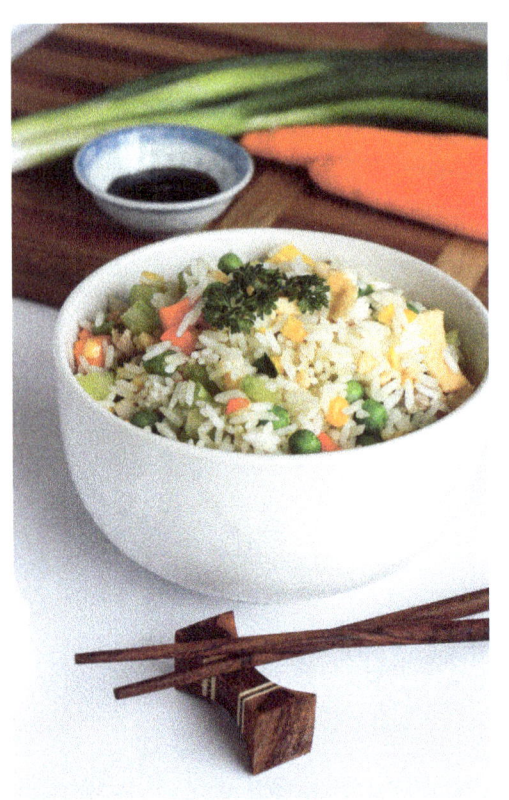
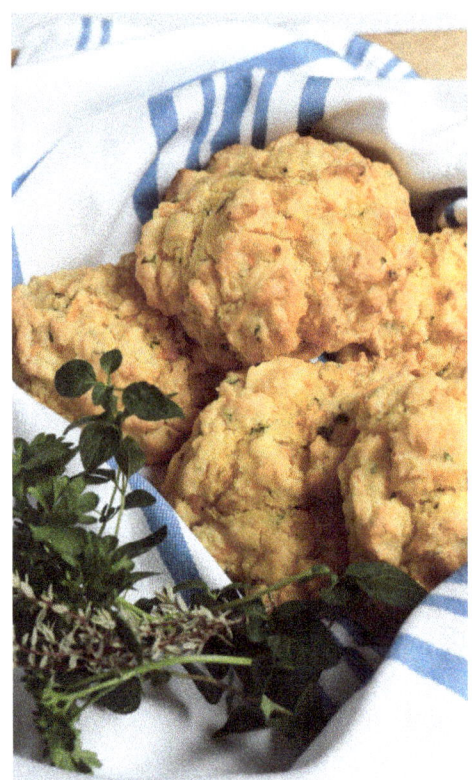
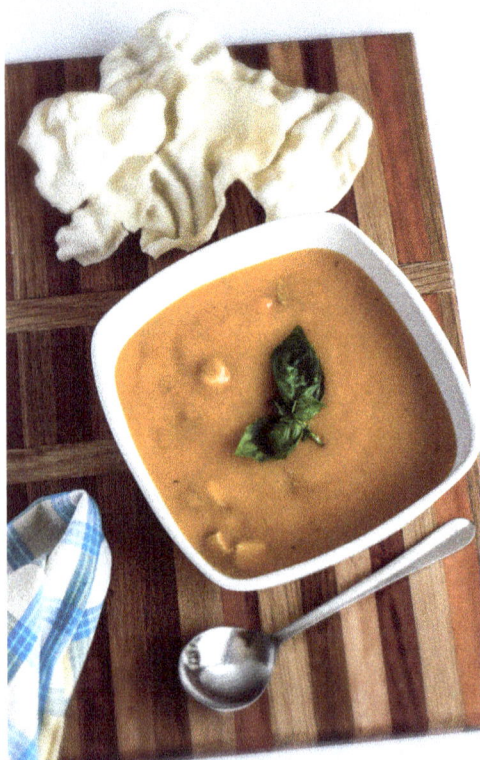
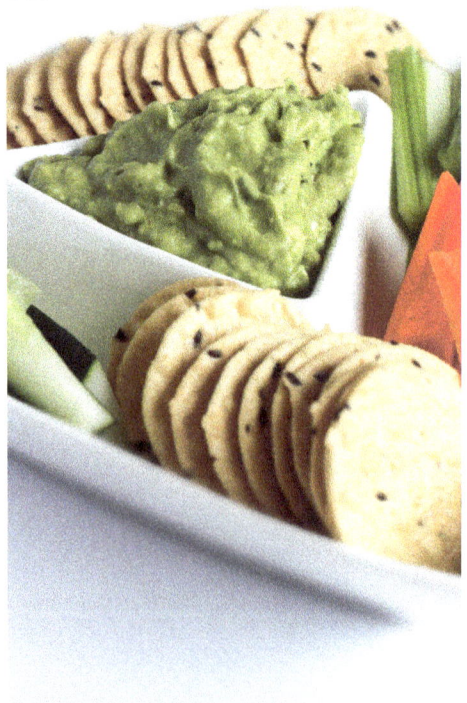

STARTERS

These are my favourite snacks or light meals, but they can also be the perfect accompaniment for any of the main dishes. They are also ideal for if you are looking for a dish to take along to a BBQ, party or just share with friends.

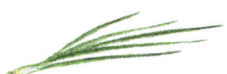

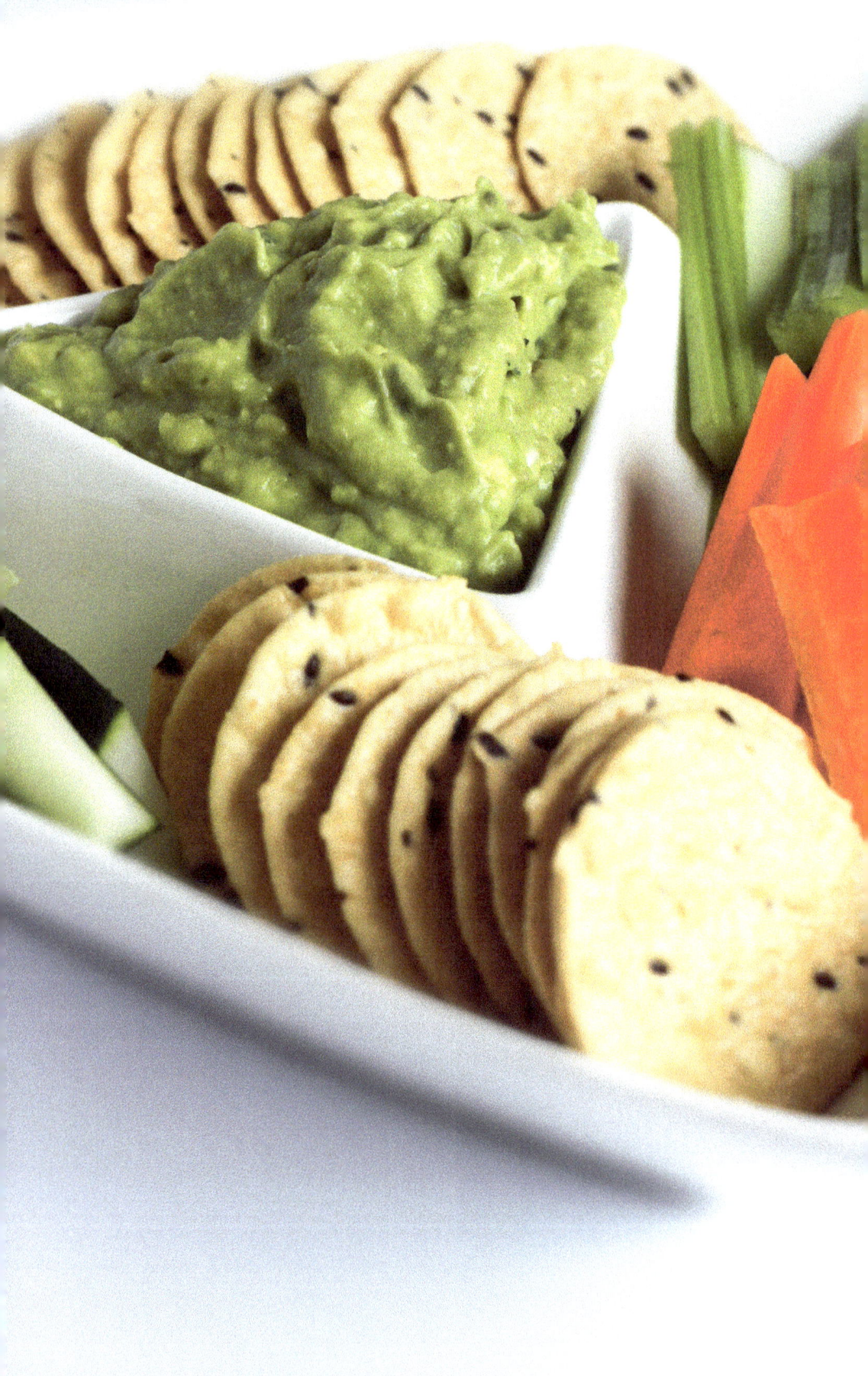

Avocado Dip

As well as a yummy dip, this recipe is very popular for people who can't have butter or margarine - it's great for a base on a sandwich. It is also a wonderful guacamole substitute but beware - it's so good, it's addictive!

INGREDIENTS
- 2 ripe (not over ripe) avocados, peeled, stoned and mashed
- 1 very finely chopped spring onion (shallot)
- 1 small clove garlic, peeled and crushed
- 2 tablespoons finely chopped fresh parsley
- ½ teaspoon sea salt
- Freshly ground pepper to taste
- 1 tablespoon lemon or lime juice
- 2 tablespoons natural soy yoghurt (or yoghurt of your choice)

METHOD
1. Mix all ingredients together and chill.
2. Serve with corn chips, rice crackers and fresh, raw vegetables.

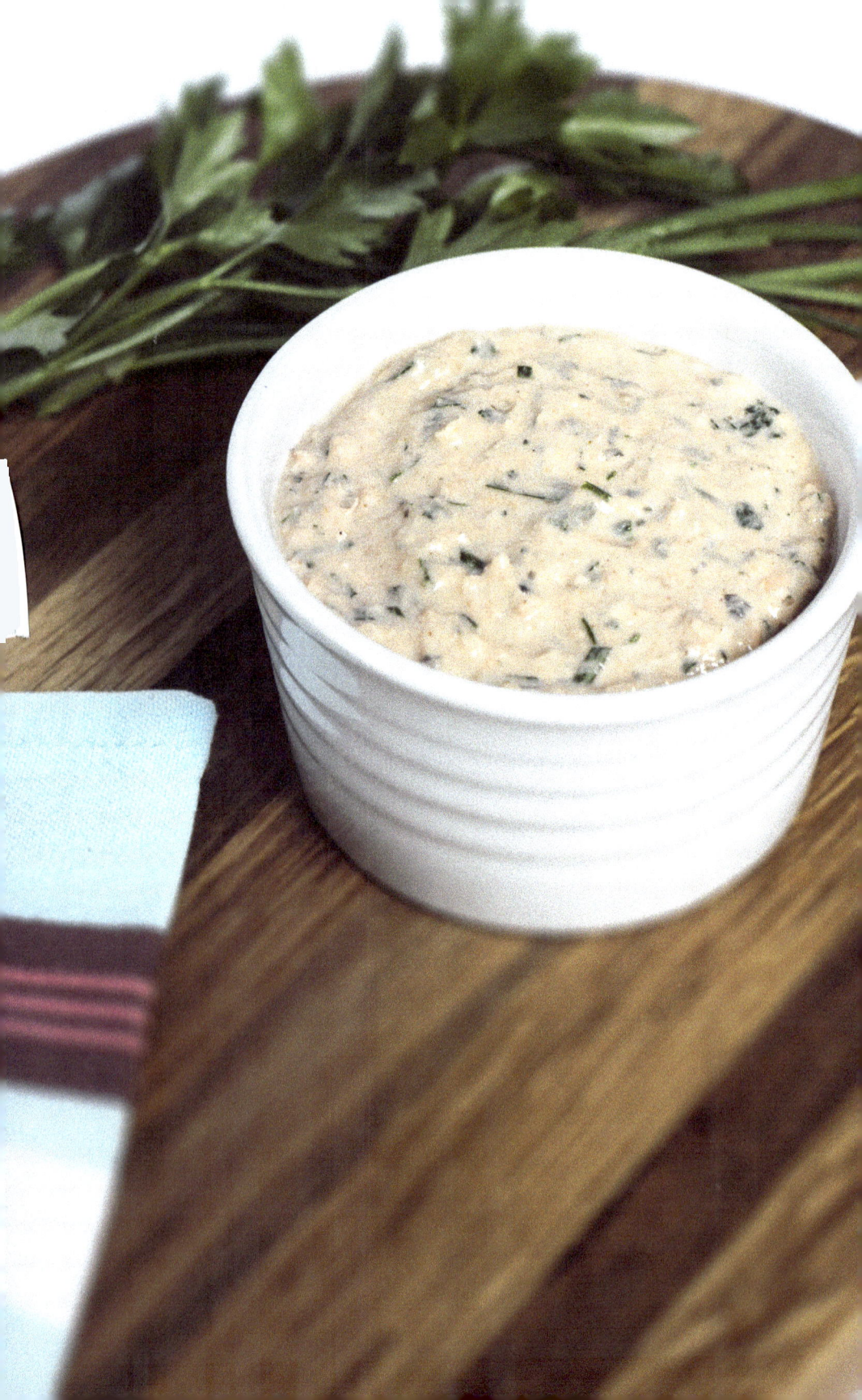

Red Salmon Dip

This dip is light and refreshing and the salmon flavour adds a really unique twist on a standard dip.

INGREDIENTS
- Small tin of red salmon (220 ml/7 oz)
- 2 tablespoons chopped fresh parsley
- ¼ teaspoon paprika
- ¼ teaspoon cayenne
- Freshly ground pepper and sea salt to taste
- ½ teaspoon lemon or lime juice
- 4 tablespoons of natural soy yoghurt (or yoghurt of your choice)

METHOD
1. Mix all the ingredients together and chill in the refrigerator.
2. Serve with rice crackers, corn chips and fresh raw vegetables.

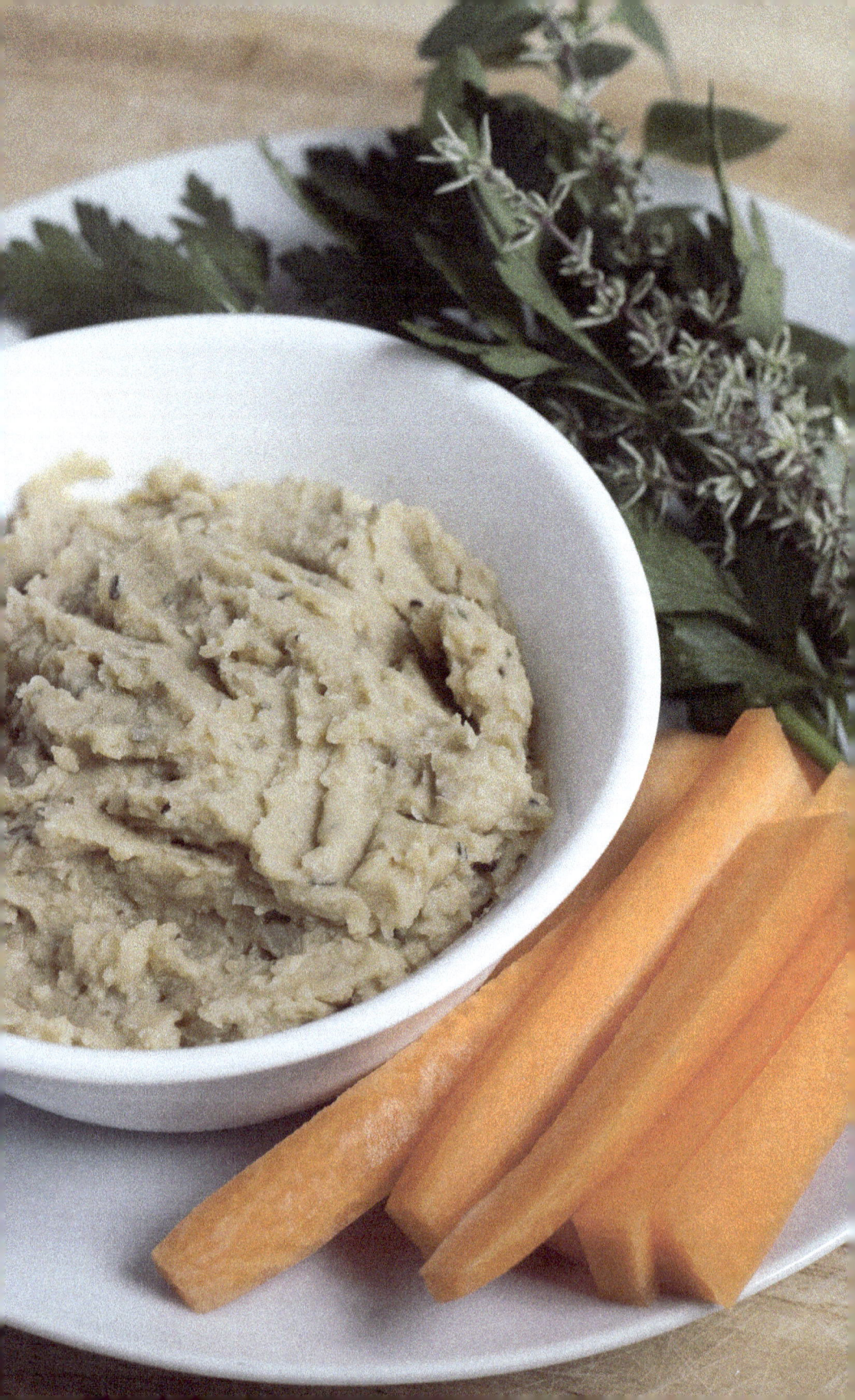

Hommus Dip

Hommus (or hummus, as some people call it) uses tahini as a key ingredient to make that lovely nutty flavour. Tahini is a paste made from ground, hulled sesame seeds and unfortunately many people have an allergy to sesame. So, my version offers the same great flavour without the risk of problems!

INGREDIENTS
- 1 can (425gm/15oz) chickpeas
- 1 clove garlic, peeled and crushed
- 2 tablespoons olive oil
- ¼ cup water
- Juice of ½ a lemon or lime
- ½ teaspoon dried rosemary
- ½ teaspoon cumin
- ½ teaspoon paprika

METHOD
1. Drain and rinse the chickpeas in cold running water.
2. Place the drained chickpeas in a blender with the garlic, lemon juice, oil, water, salt, rosemary, cumin and paprika.
3. Blend until smooth, add more oil if necessary.

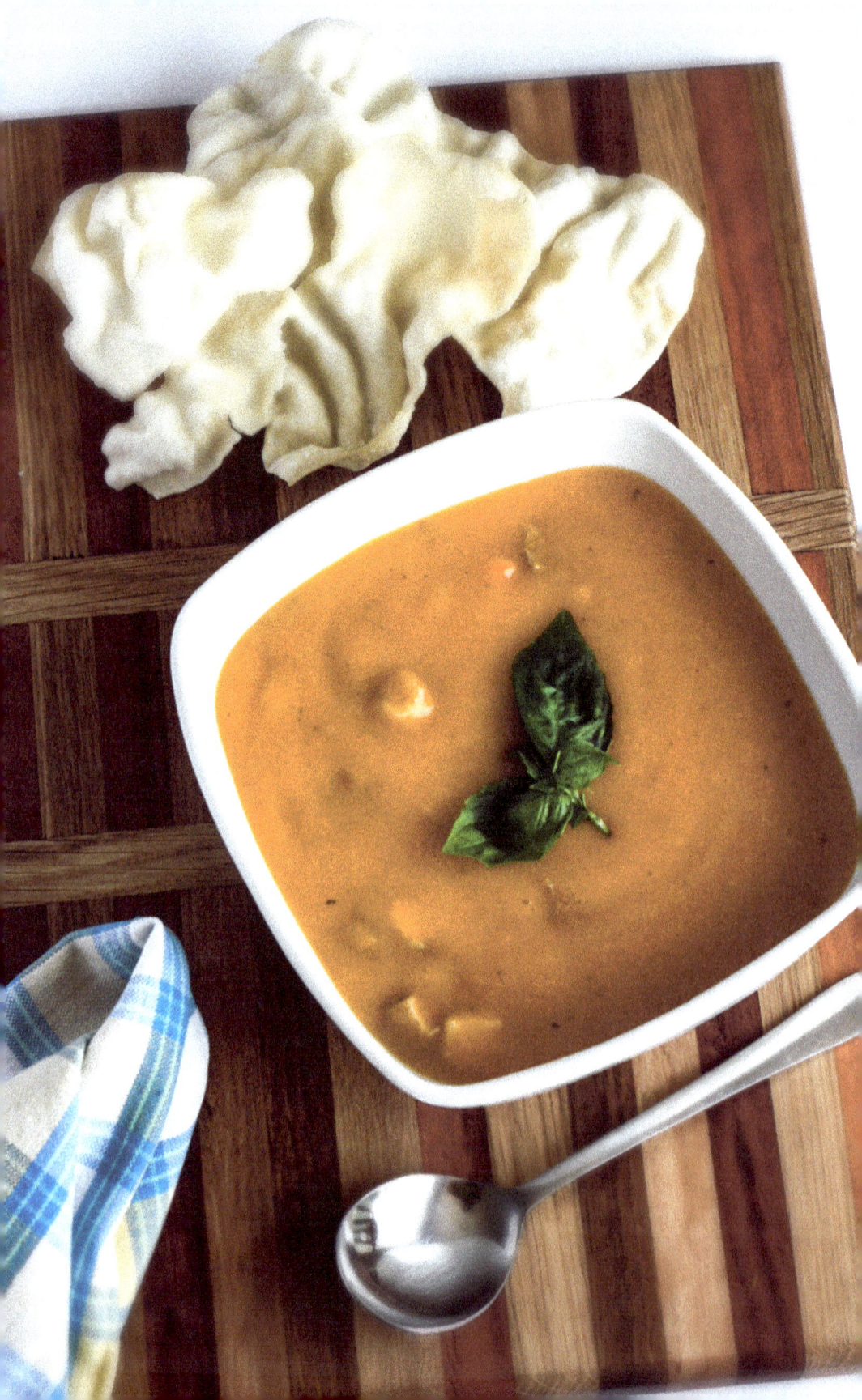

Chunky Pork Soup

This recipe is equally as tasty without the pork and made with veggie stock as a vegetarian option. It's a lovely, chunky soup and is beautifully filling on a cold winter's day.

INGREDIENTS
- 600gm (21 oz) pork spare ribs
- 1 clove garlic, peeled and finely chopped
- 2 cups pumpkin, peeled and cut into chunks
- 1 large onion, peeled and diced
- 1 cup carrots, peeled and sliced
- 1 cup potato, peeled and cut into chunks
- 1 cup celery diced
- 1 tablespoon arrowroot
- 4 cups chicken stock
- 1 tablespoon fresh parsley, scissor cut
- 1 tablespoon fresh basil, scissor cut
- 1 teaspoon sea salt
- 1 teaspoon freshly ground pepper

METHOD
1. Fry pork in frying pan until cooked.
2. Remove meat from pan and refrigerate for later use.
3. Add vegetables into meat oil and toss until onion is transparent (approx. 5 minutes).
4. Remove vegetables from pan and put into large saucepan.
5. Add arrowroot and stir through vegetables.
6. Add stock, parsley, basil, salt and pepper and stir through.
7. Bring to boil then lower heat and cook for a further 30 minutes or until vegetables are soft.
8. Cut all fat and bones from spare ribs and discard.
9. Cut meat into small cubes and put back in refrigerator.
10. Remove soup from stove.
11. Process, puree or blend vegetables, leaving some vegetables whole for chunky texture.
12. Add meat and reheat.

Serve with a spoonful of yoghurt, topped with fresh chives and black pepper.

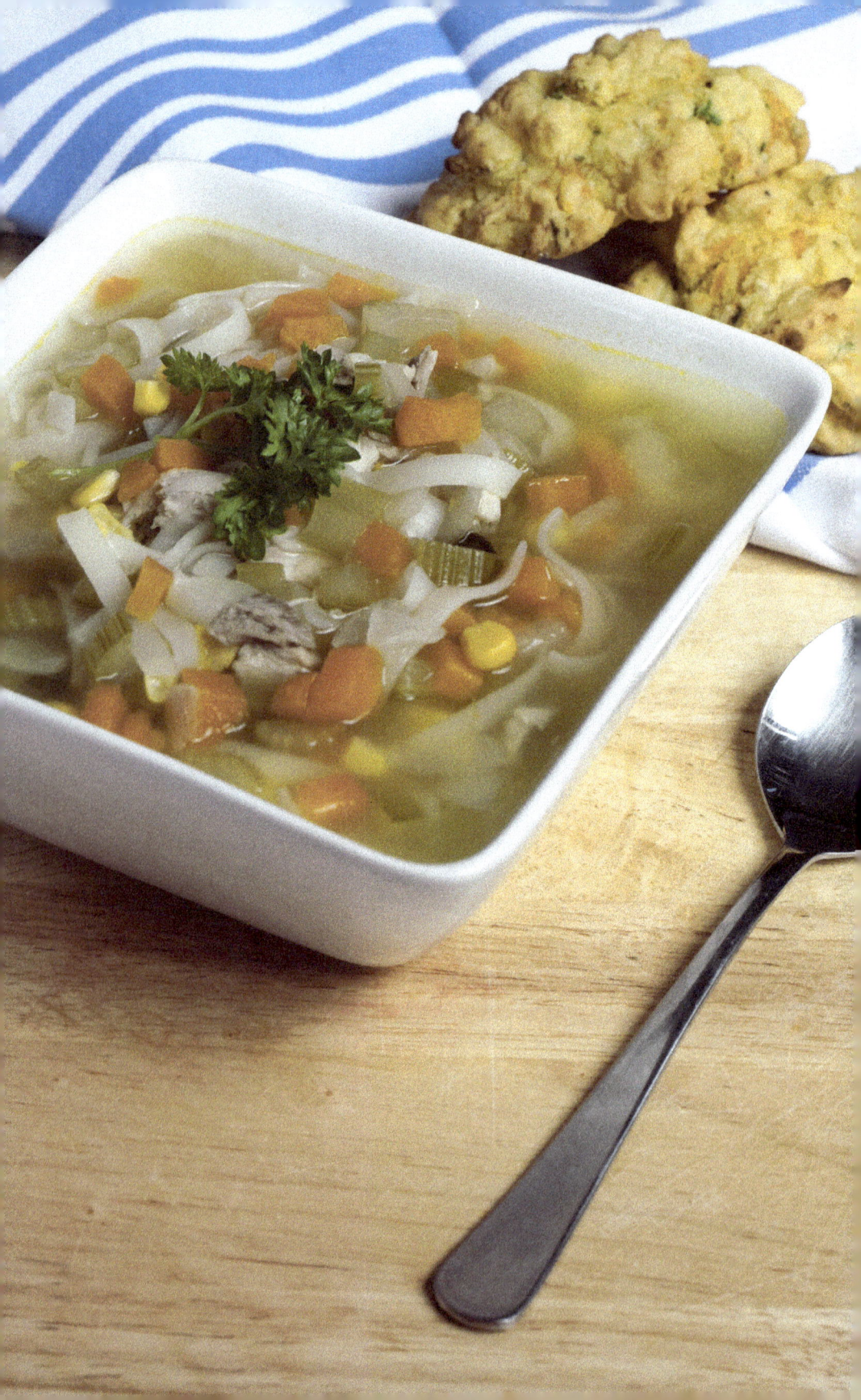

Chicken Soup

Both children and adults love this soup and it is fabulous if you are feeling a bit run down or have the flu. The rice noodles turn it from a broth into a more substantial soup - so feel free to leave them out if you'd like something lighter.

INGREDIENTS
- 8 cups chicken stock
- 1 large onion peeled and diced
- 2 medium carrots peeled and diced
- 1 large stalk of celery diced
- 1 tablespoon celery leaves, finely chopped
- 1 tablespoon fresh parsley, finely chopped
- ½ teaspoon sea salt
- Freshly ground black pepper to taste
- 1 cup of cooked, free-range chicken pieces, roughly chopped
- 2 cups of broken rice sticks

METHOD
1. In a large pot add the chicken stock, vegetables, salt, parsley and celery leaves.
2. Bring them to the boil and then simmer for 40 minutes.
3. Ten minutes before serving add the chicken pieces and broken rice sticks.

Season with ground pepper and serve with savoury scones (see page 55).

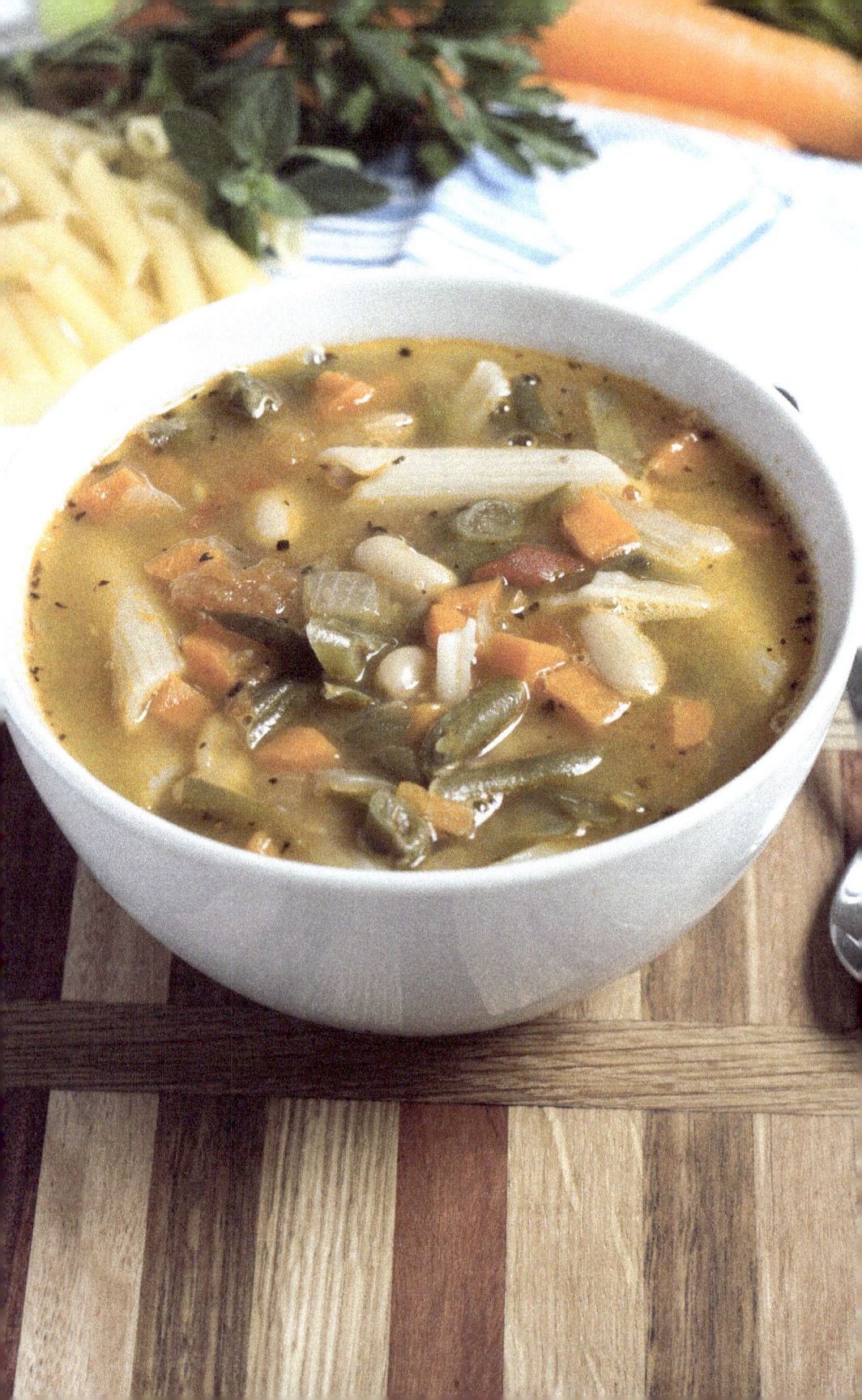

Minestrone

One of the greatest complaints many people with food allergies have is that they are often hungry. A high protein diet can definitely do that to you and if you can't eat dairy either, or you are vegetarian, it can limit your options even more. This soup, though, is healthy, easy, tasty and will fill you up!

INGREDIENTS
- 8 cups of vegetable stock (see page 35)
- 2 tablespoons extra virgin olive oil
- 3 clove garlics crushed
- 1 large onion diced
- 2 stalks celery diced
- 1 large carrot diced
- 1 ½ cups green beans sliced
- 1 small zucchini diced
- 1 x 400gm (13oz) tin of low sodium cannellini beans, drained and rinsed
- 4 fresh tomatoes (skinned and diced) or 1 x 400gm (13oz) tin of low sodium crushed tomatoes
- 1 tablespoon fresh oregano finely diced
- 1 tablespoon fresh thyme finely diced
- 1 tablespoon fresh basil finely diced
- 1 tablespoon fresh parsley finely diced
- Sea salt and freshly ground pepper to taste
- 1 cup of gluten-free pasta (I have used penne)

METHOD
1. Heat the oil in a large pot over medium to high heat, add the onion and garlic cloves and cook until the onion is transparent.
2. Add stock and bring to the boil then add the carrots and green beans.
3. Reduce the heat and add the celery and zucchini and simmer until the zucchini is soft.
4. Add herbs, salt, pepper, tomatoes, pasta and cannellini beans, bring to the boil then simmer until the pasta is cooked.

Top with fresh basil when serving.

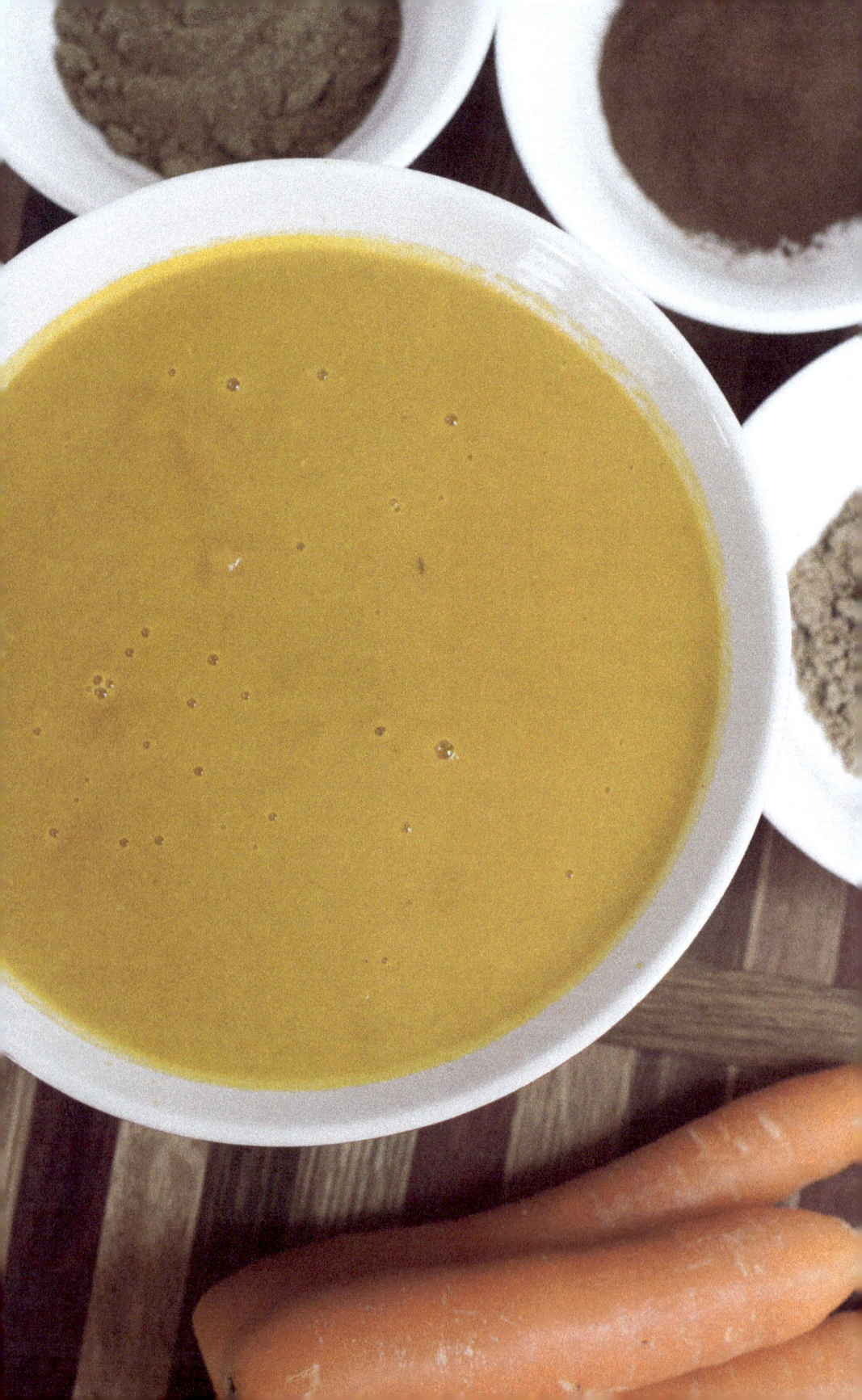

Spicy Carrot Soup

This is another great vegetarian option and I love this because I am big fan of spicy flavours - they warm you right down to your toes. If you don't like things with quite so much kick, just halve your measures of cumin and paprika.

INGREDIENTS
- 6 cups of vegetable stock (see page 37)
- 2 tablespoons olive oil
- 1 large onion, peeled and diced
- 1 medium potato, peeled and sliced
- 3 cups carrots, peeled and sliced
- 1 teaspoon ground coriander
- 1 teaspoon cumin
- 1 teaspoon paprika
- Sea salt and ground black pepper to taste

METHOD
1. Heat oil, over medium heat, in a large saucepan. Add carrot, onions and potato and cook gently until onions become transparent.
2. Add the spices and cook for one minute stirring all the time.
3. Add the stock, bring to the boil then cover and simmer until the carrots are tender (approximately 45 minutes).
4. Cool the soup then place in a blender or food processor and puree.
5. Put the soup back into the saucepan and reheat, season to taste with salt and pepper.

Serve with thyme and garlic flatbread (see page 57).

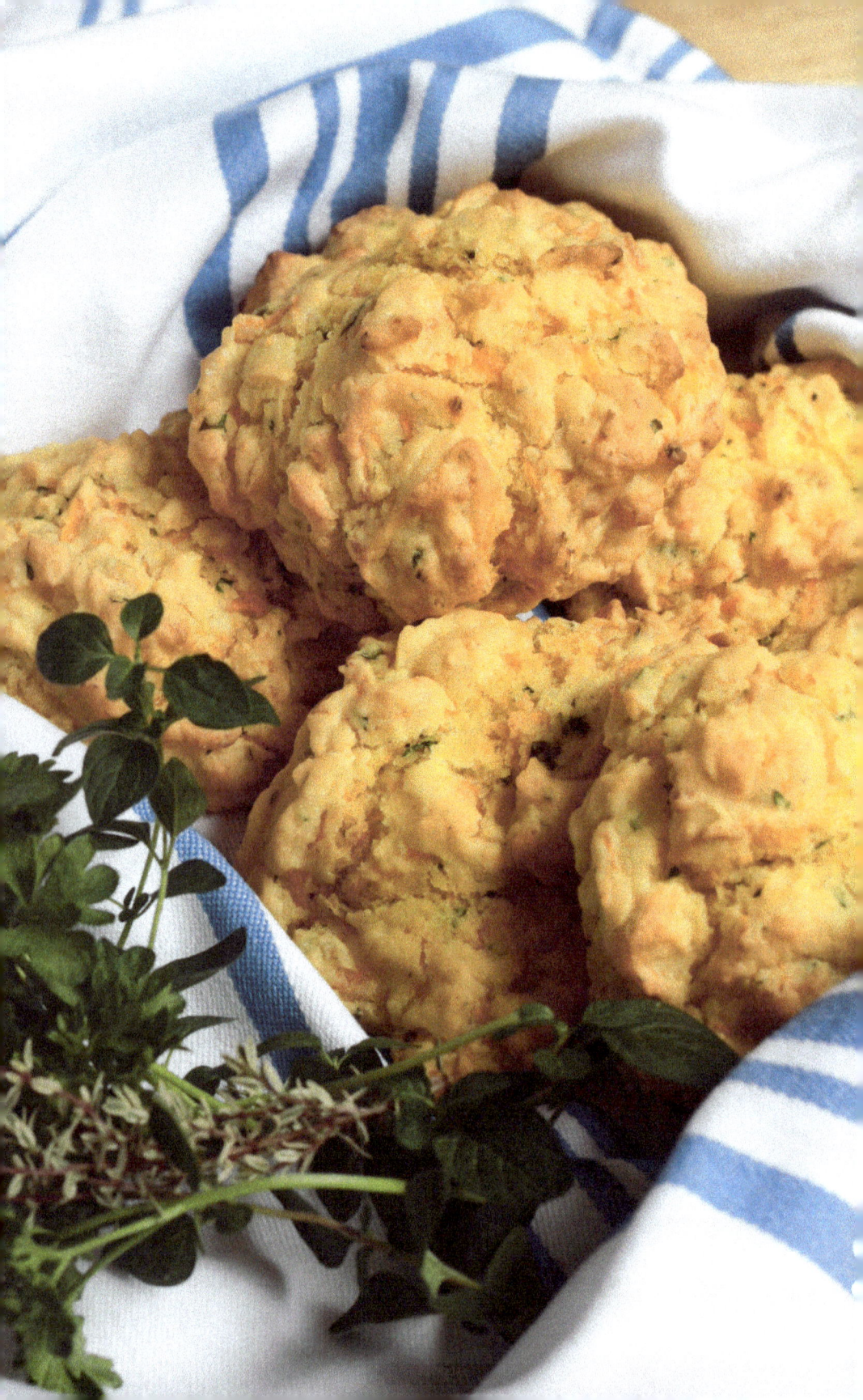

Savoury Scones

These are a family favourite and when I could no longer have cheese, I thought it was the end of this recipe in my life! I am happy to report that this version not only tastes just as good, but it's just as easy to make as well.

INGREDIENTS
- 5 tablespoons olive oil
- 1 ¼ cups rice milk
- 3 cups gluten-free self raising flour
- ½ teaspoon sea salt
- 1 large onion peeled and grated
- 1 large carrot peeled and grated
- 1 cup grated pumpkin
- 1 tablespoon finely chopped fresh parsley
- 1 tablespoon finely chopped fresh basil
- 1-2 tablespoons of finely chopped fresh mixed herbs (eg. rosemary, thyme, marjoram, oregano, sage, tarragon)
- Freshly cracked black pepper to taste

METHOD
1. Pre-heat oven to 200 degrees C (or 380 degrees F).
2. Sift flour and salt into a large bowl.
3. Make a well in the centre of dry ingredients and add oil and milk and mix.
4. Add grated vegetables and herbs and stir or use your hands and work them into the mixture.
5. Season with cracked pepper.
6. Lightly grease oven trays with olive oil.
7. Place a dessertspoonful of mixture on tray – leaving room for scones to spread.
8. Place trays in oven for 15-20 minutes or until golden and cooked through.
9. Take the scones out of the oven and wrap in a cotton tea towel to keep warm and fresh before serving.

Makes approximately 15 scones depending on the size.

Serve scones hot or cold, whole or halved topped with your favourite spread.

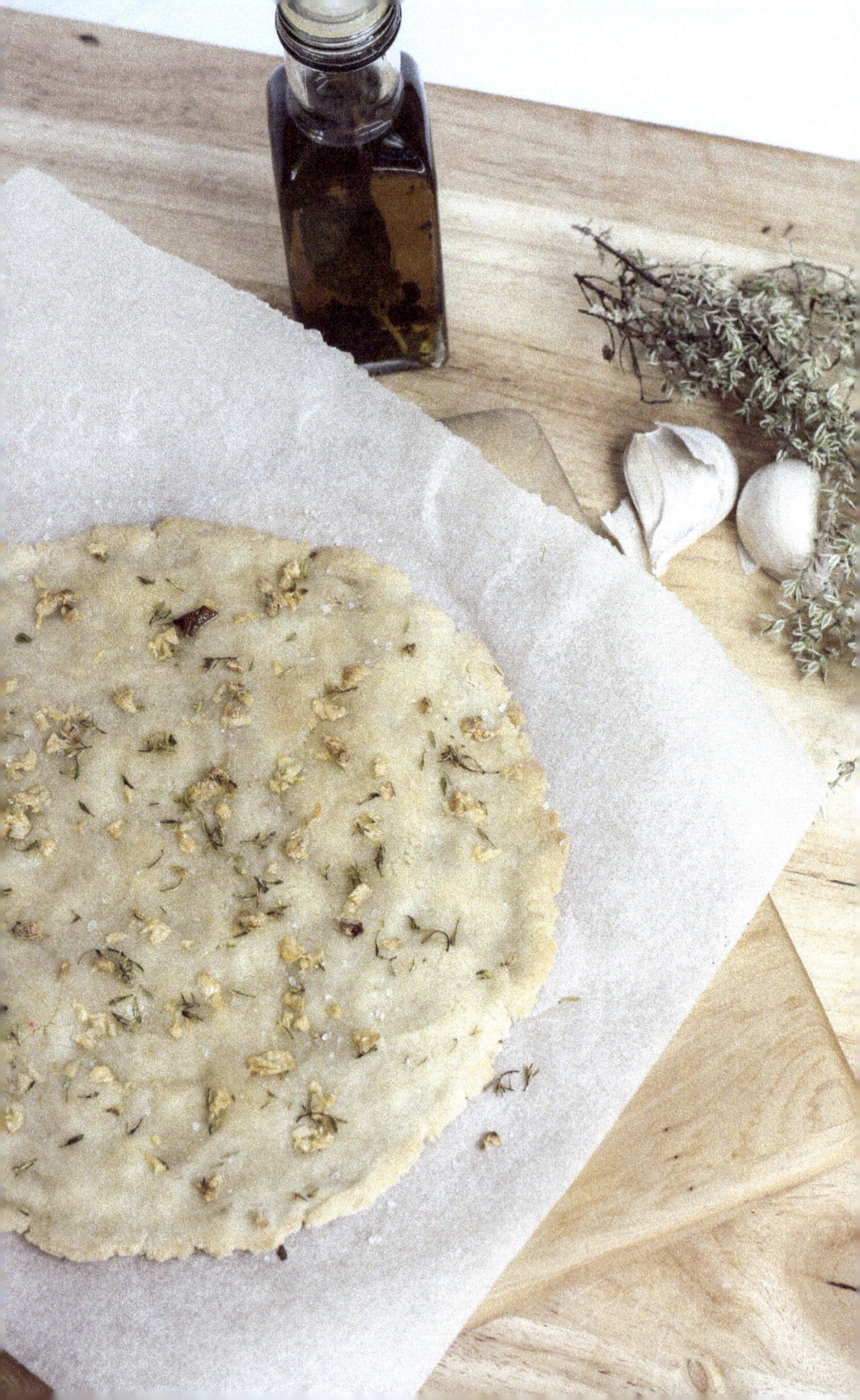

Thyme Flatbread

Anyone on a gluten-free or yeast-free diet misses bread terribly. When I first made this, I was actually amazed at how nice this was and it was lovely to have a tasty flat bread that was filled with flavour. A great accompaniment for soups and stews, or just nice as a light snack.

INGREDIENTS
- 1 ½ cups plain gluten-free plain flour
- ½ teaspoon sea salt
- ½ cup rice milk
- ¼ cup olive or sunflower oil
- 1 egg, beaten
- 1 teaspoon fresh thyme, finely chopped
- 2 clove garlics, peeled and crushed
- Herbed oil (see page 23) and sea salt to garnish

METHOD
1. Pre-heat oven to 200 degrees C (400 degrees F).
2. Combine flour and salt in a bowl and mix, make a well in the centre.
3. Pour rice milk and oil into the well and mix until combined.
4. Add beaten egg and mix until you make a dough that forms into a ball.
5. Place baking paper onto a pizza tray and spread mixture with your hands onto the baking paper, pushing it out with your fingertips to form a circle the size of the pizza tray.
6. Sprinkle on the thyme and garlic.
7. Bake until golden and crispy (approximately 10 to 12 minutes).
7. Remove from oven and put flatbread onto a serving plate. While still warm, drizzle with herbed oil and sea salt to garnish.

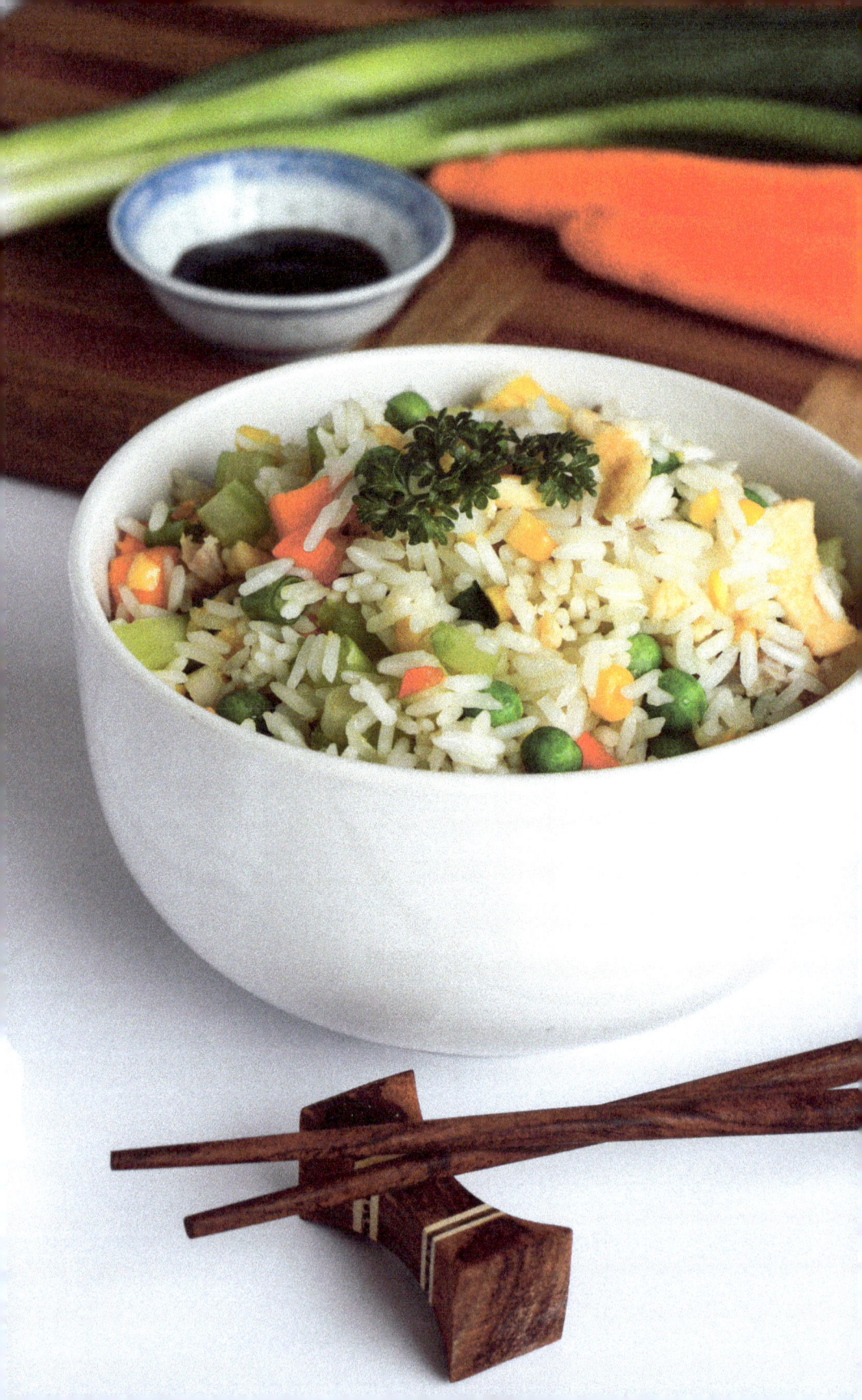

Fried Rice

My fried rice has become a family favourite over the years. It can be a meal on its own, as an accompaniment with a BBQ, as a side if you are cooking an Asian themed spread and it can also be delicious served cold like a salad. The beauty of it is that you can use any vegetables or meats that you have on hand to flavour.

INGREDIENTS
- 3 cups cooked rice (completely cold, and kept in the refrigerator until required)
- 3 eggs, beaten
- 3 tablespoons olive oil
- Juice of 1 lime or lemon
- ½ cup chopped spring onions (scallions)
- ½ cup carrots, chopped finely
- ½ cup capsicum (pepper) chopped finely
- ½ cup cooked corn cornels
- ½ cup cooked peas
- Salt and pepper to taste

METHOD
1. Heat 1 tablespoon of olive oil in a frying pan.
2. Pour in beaten eggs to cover bottom of pan.
3. Cook until mixture is ready to flip over and quickly cook the other side.
4. Remove egg – cut into small squares and keep aside.
5. Add 2 tablespoons of oil in the wok (or large frypan), heat, then add cold rice and toss through.
6. Add vegetables and lime (lemon juice) and mix through.

Wheat-free soy sauce and cooked diced meat (pork, chicken, seafood) can be added for extra flavour.

1 ½ cups of raw rice make approximately 3 cups of cooked rice.

Pre-cook the rice the day before (or at least three hours before) to allow the rice to completely cool in the refrigerator (this will ensure the rice isn't 'sticky' when you're combining the ingredients.

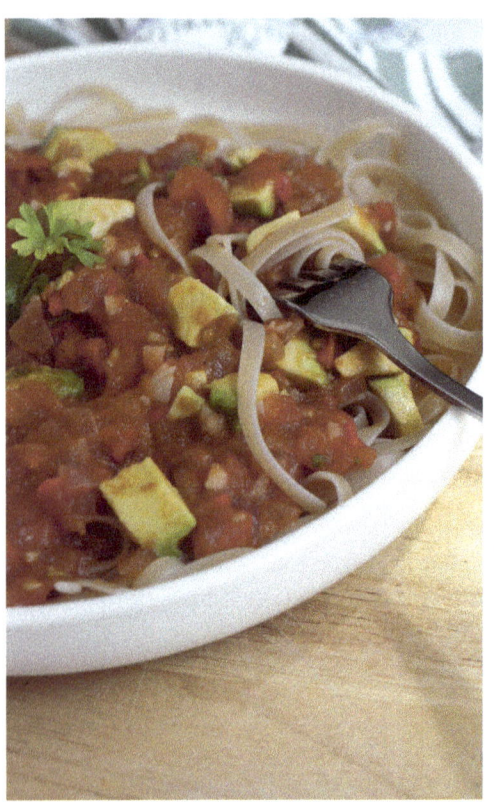
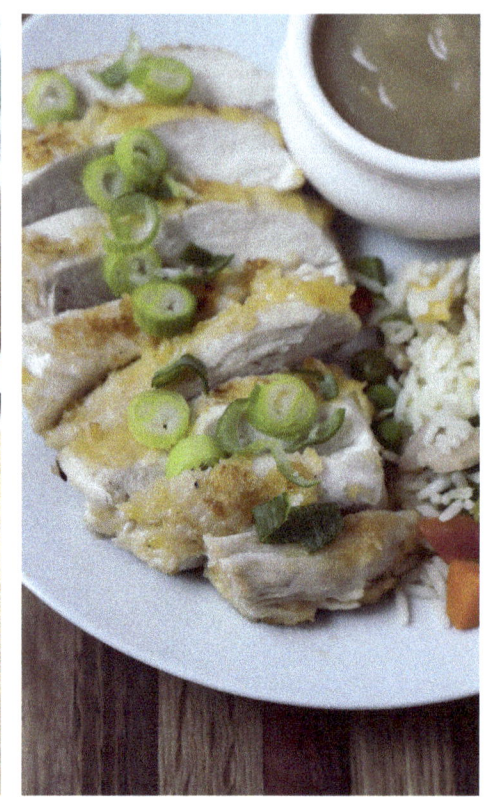
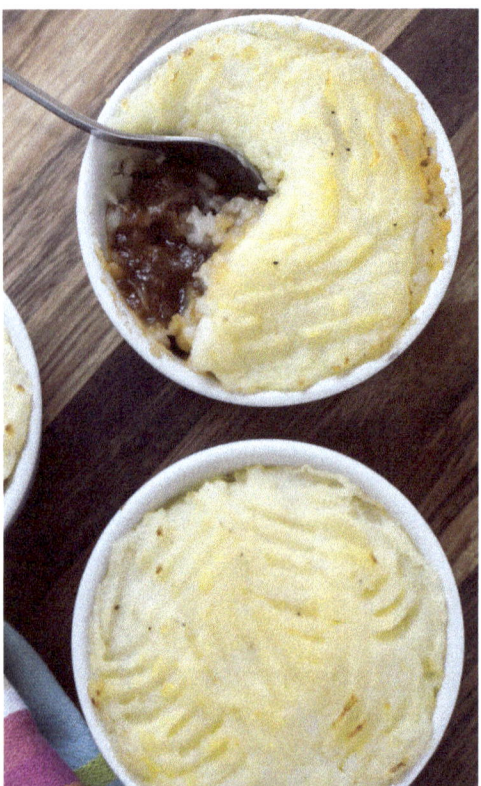
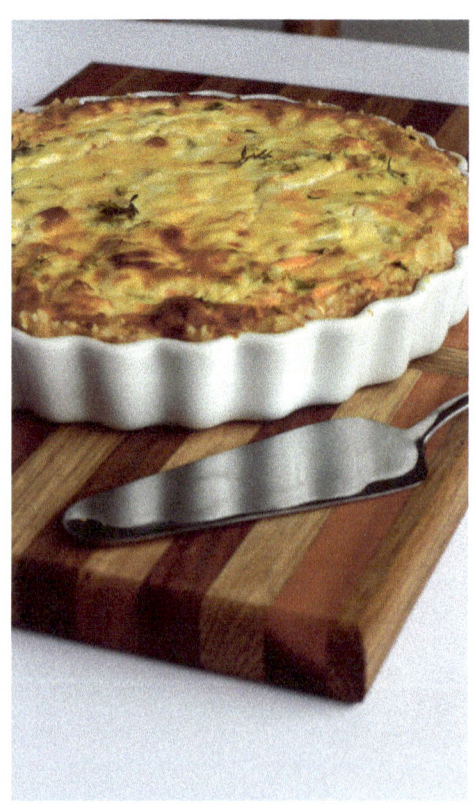

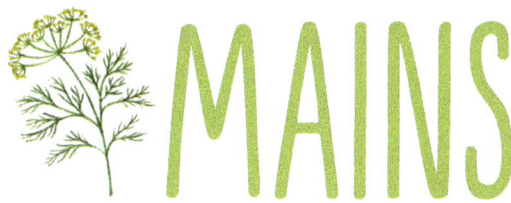
MAINS

Great tasting and filling meals that have been developed to accomodate all ages and all taste buds! Ideally, you are then only cooking one meal for all family members or friends - regardless of their dietary requirements. All of my mains are all quick, easy and simple to make but (most importantly) they taste delicious!

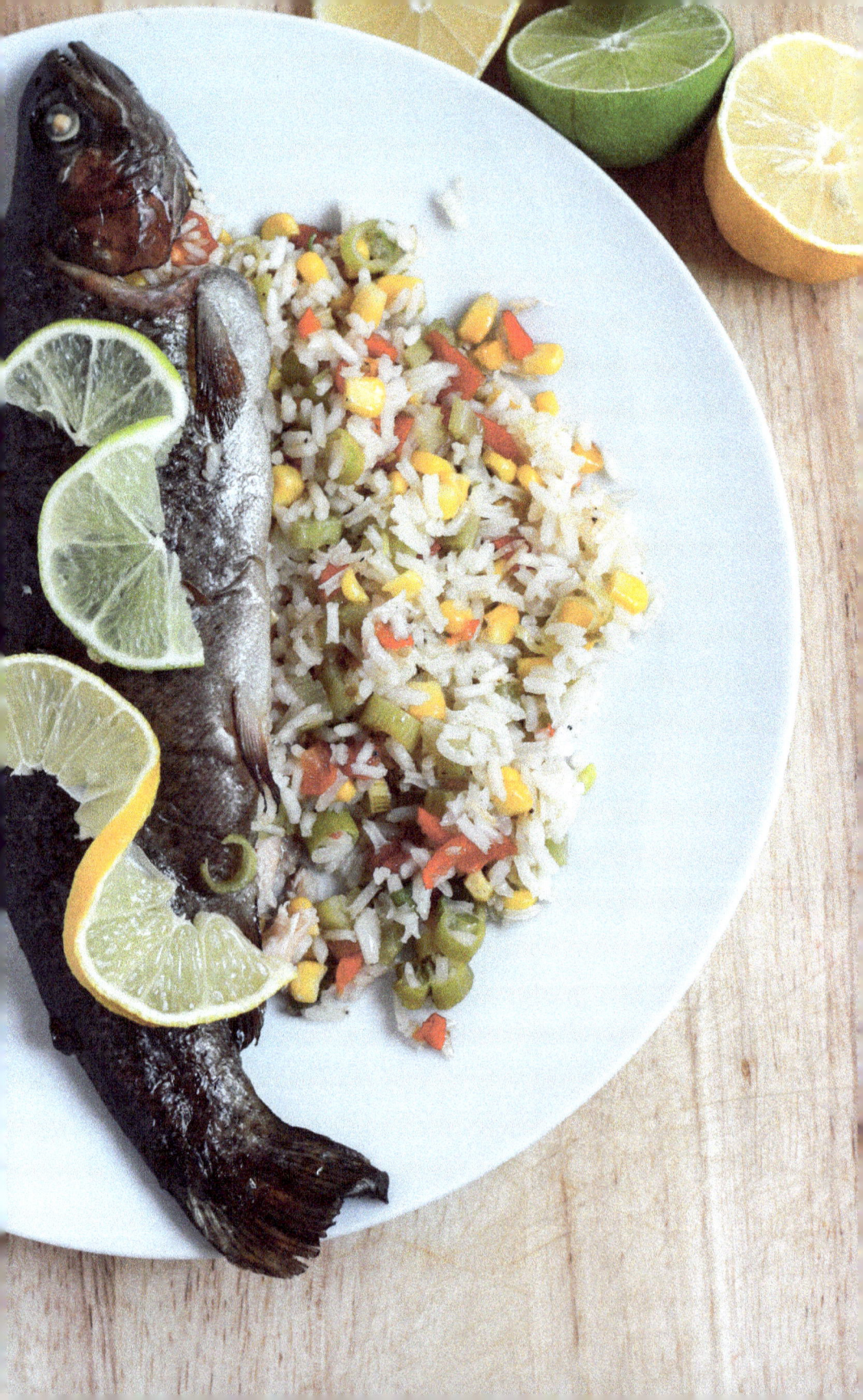

Stuffed Rainbow Trout

This is a really simple dish - the filling becomes the side dishes - so you have no extras to prepare and, even better, no dishes! The vegetables give the fish a great flavour and baking the fish makes it soft and melt in your mouth.

INGREDIENTS
- 4 rainbow trout
- 2 cups long grain white rice
- 3 spring onions (shallots) finely diced
- ¼ cup capsicum (bell pepper) finely diced
- ¼ cup cooked corn kernels
- ¼ cup celery, finely diced
- 2 tablespoons finely chopped fresh parsley
- 1 tomato, finely diced
- Olive oil or vegan spread
- Sea salt and freshly ground black pepper to taste
- aluminium foil for wrapping fish

METHOD
1. Pre-heat oven 180 degrees C or 350 degrees F.
2. Cook rice just until grains separate – do not overcook.
3. Drain the rice, rinse with cold water then drain well.
4. Add vegetables to rice, season with salt and pepper and mix with oil or vegan spread.
5. Cut 4 large pieces of foil, large enough to wrap each piece of fish in.
6. Grease each piece of foil with oil or vegan spread.
7. Place each fish in the centre of a piece of foil.
8. Fill fish cavity with rice mixture.
9. Place small dobs of vegan spread on each fish or brush with oil.
10. Wrap foil around fish like a parcel.
11. Cook in a moderate oven for 30 minutes.
12. Remove from foil to serve.

Serves 4

*A word on fish: many people are a little scared of fish. Perhaps they didn't grow up eating it, or they had a bad experience once. It's a wonderful, healthy and easy meat though so I encourage you to try this recipe as a great starter. Just ask your local fishmonger or deli worker for the full fish. It will have been gutted, but not filleted so there are still bones in there. They bake so beautifully though, the meat literally peels away from the bones. The smaller the fish, however, the more bones you are likely to encounter.

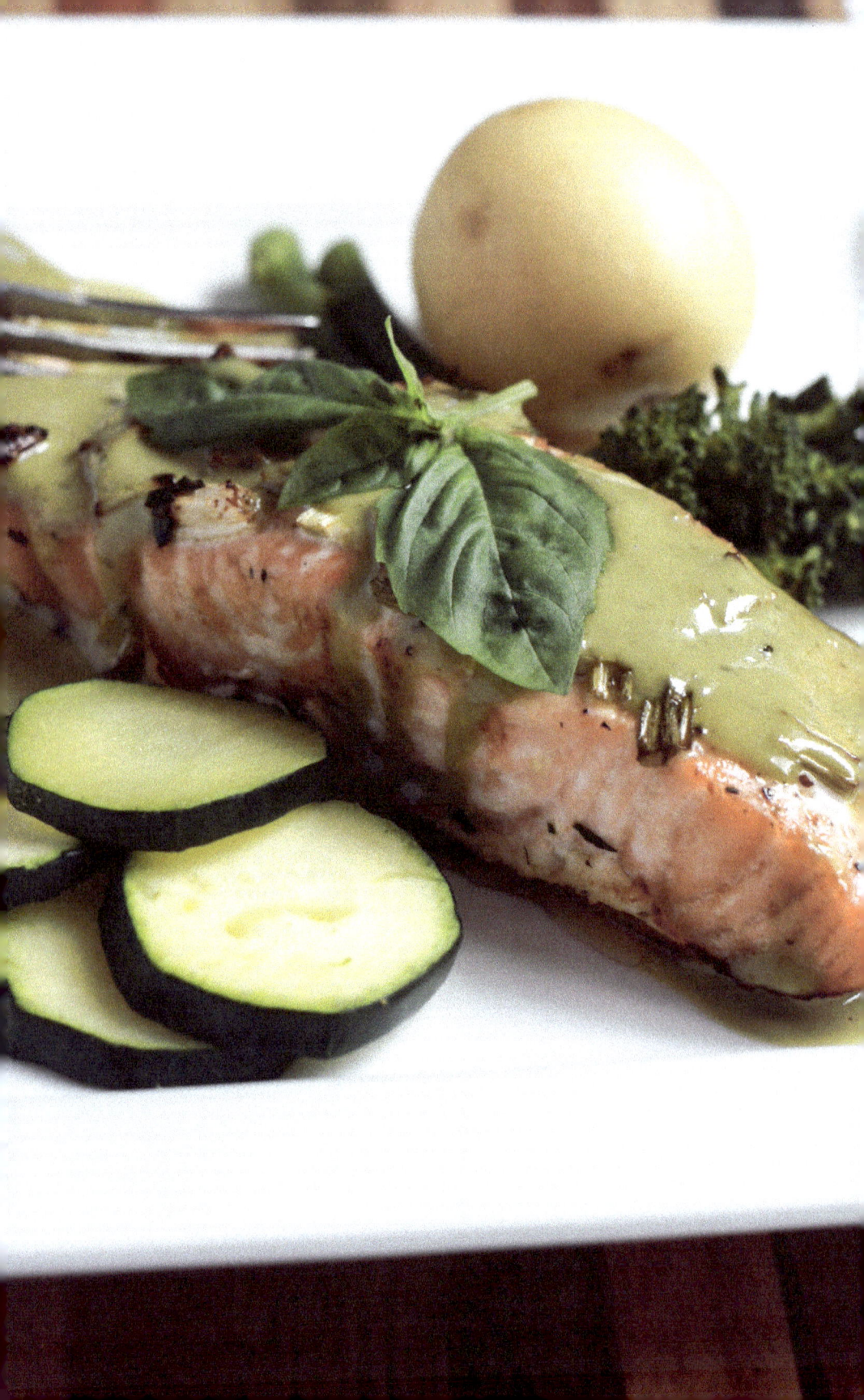

Baked Fish Steaks

This is a very, very easy recipe - both to make and to digest. It is perfect for a dinner party too...even non-fish lovers tend to find salmon appealing. It's delicious and it looks lovely too.

INGREDIENTS
- 4 Atlantic salmon steaks
- Olive oil
- 1 lemon or lime
- 3 spring onions (shallots)
- Fresh parsley
- Fresh basil leaves

METHOD
1. Pre-heat oven to 160 degrees C or 320 degrees F.
2. Grease a baking dish with olive oil.
3. Place fish steaks in a oven proof dish.
4. Squeeze lemon juice over the fish, and sprinkle with salt and pepper.
5. Cut parsley and spring onions (shallots) with scissors and scatter over each steak.
6. Drizzle Basil and Sun Dried Tomato Oil (see page 27) over the top of each fish steak and then sprinkle with basil leaves.
7. Cover with foil and bake in a moderate oven for 20 minutes.

Serve with Basil and Anchovy Sauce (see page 33) and steamed vegetables.

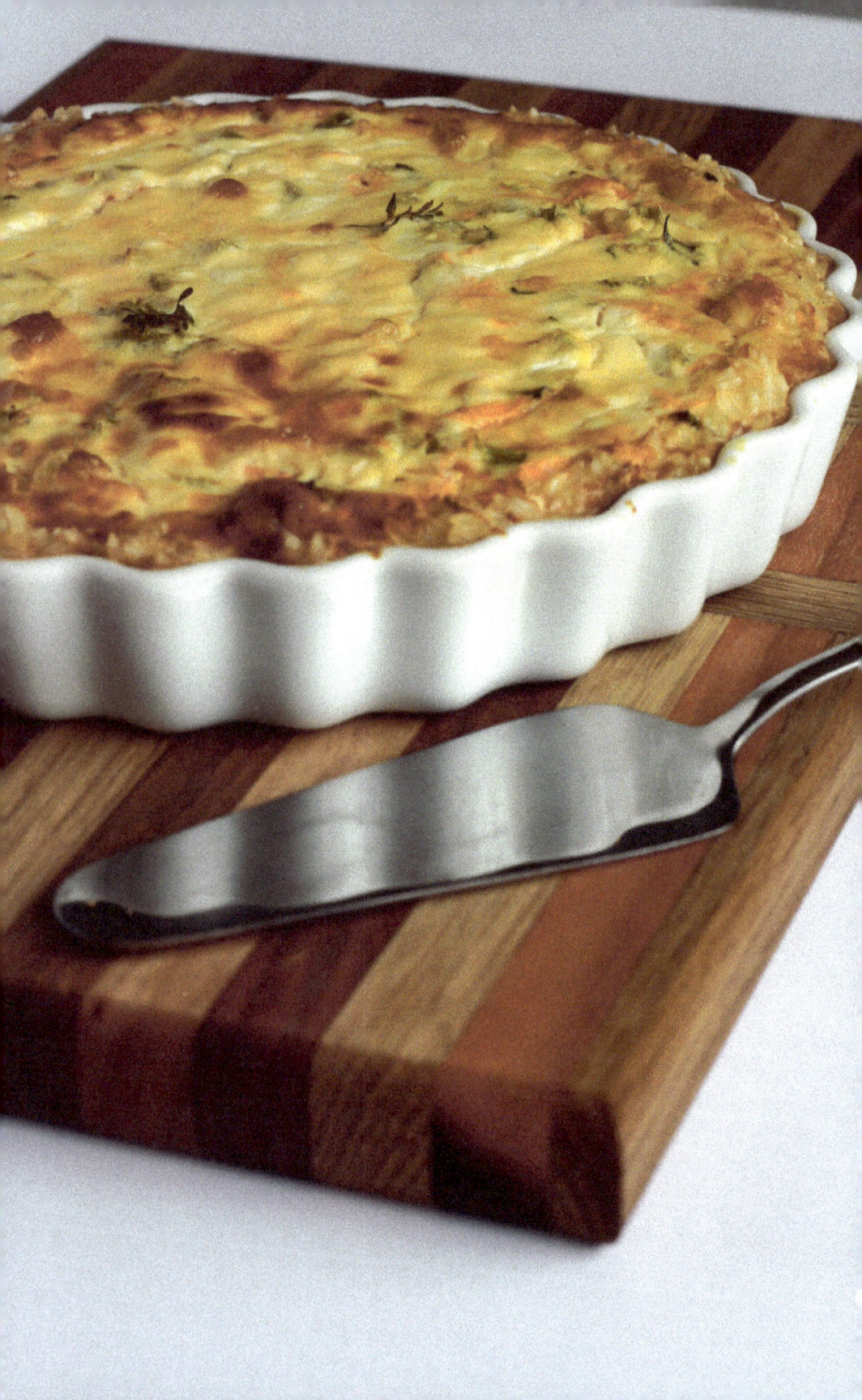

Red Salmon Pie

The thing that is a struggle for many people with dairy allergies or intolerances is not being able to cook with cheese. And those eating gluten-free will often complain about missing out on a yummy pie. When I couldn't have cheese anymore I found the combination of egg, soy milk and yoghurt both set and tasted like cheese - perfect!

INGREDIENTS

Pie Shell:
- 2 cups cooked rice
- ½ cup chopped spring onions (scallions)
- 1 egg
- ½ tablespoon olive oil
- Sea salt and ground black pepper to taste

Filling:
- 210gm or (7oz) tin of red salmon
- 2 beaten eggs
- 4 tablespoons of natural soy yoghurt (or yoghurt of your choice)
- ¾ cup of malt-free, sugar-free soy milk (or milk or your choice)
- Sea salt and ground black pepper to taste
- ¼ teaspoon of dry mustard
- ¼ cup grated carrot
- ¼ cup finely diced celery
- 1 tablespoon chopped parsley
- 1 tablespoon chopped chives

METHOD

Pre-heat your oven to 180 degrees C (350 degrees F).

Pie Shell:
1. Mix rice, spring onions, beaten egg and oil together in a bowl. Season to taste with salt and pepper.
2. Lightly grease with oil, a flan or pie dish.
3. Press rice mixture onto the base and up the sides of the dish.

Filling:
1. Drain the tin of red salmon, reserve the liquid and keep in a bowl.
2. Mash the salmon, bones included and spoon over the base of the pie shell.
3. Place the carrot, celery and chives on top of salmon.
4. Combine the eggs, mustard, salmon liquid, milk, yoghurt and salt and pepper, and pour over the salmon, carrot, celery and chives.

Bake the pie in a moderate oven, for approximately one hour or until the top is firm.

Vegetables of your choice can be used in the pie eg. Chopped tomatoes and peppers (capsicum).

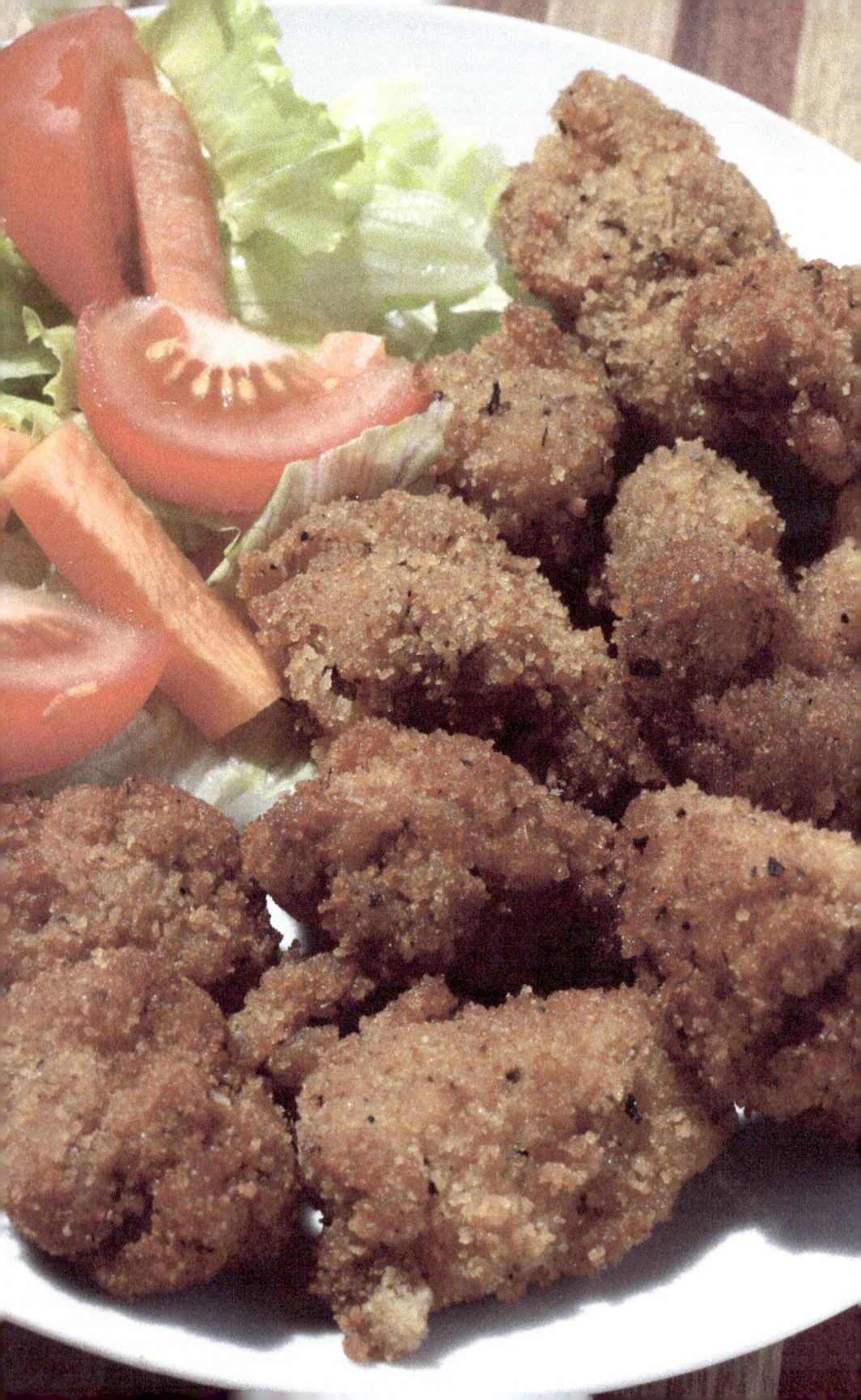

Chicken Nuggets

When you have a restricted diet, takeaway is definitely off the menu. My grandkids are often a bit confused as to why I can't eat 'junk' food. These are the perfect chicken nugget alternative - healthy, tasty and easy to make - and the kids love them too!

INGREDIENTS
- 750gm (1 Ib 8 oz) free range organic, skinned chicken breasts
- 3 tablespoons gluten-free cornflour
- 1 egg (beaten)
- 1 cup gluten-free breadcrumbs
- Oil for frying

Herb and spice mix:
- ½ teaspoon ground black pepper
- ½ teaspoon sea salt
- ½ teaspoon paprika
- ½ teaspoon onion powder
- ½ teaspoon garlic salt
- 1 teaspoon mustard powder
- 1 teaspoon ginger powder
- ¼ teaspoon dried thyme
- ¼ teaspoon dried oregano
- ½ teaspoon dried basil

METHOD
1. Pre-heat oven to 100 degrees C (212 degrees F).
2. Halve the chicken breasts and then cut the chicken into nugget shapes or bite size pieces.
3. Put the chicken pieces into a large bowl.
4. Put all the ingredients for the herb and spice mix into a small bowl and mix well.
5. Add the herb and spice mixture into the chicken pieces and stir through until well coated.
6. Pour the beaten egg into the mix and stir though.
7. Add the cornflour and mix well.
8. Lastly add the breadcrumbs and stir through until well covered.
9. Set aside for 5 to 10 minutes.
10. Fill a deep cooker with enough oil to come halfway up the sides. Bring the oil up to hot, over medium-hot heat but not smoking.
11. Put enough chicken shapes into the oil without over crowding it.
12. Deep fry until the outside of the chicken nugget is golden brown and the chicken is tender, about 5 minutes.
13. Remove pieces as they are done, drain well and place on a wire rack set in an oven tray and keep the chicken warm in the oven until all the pieces are cooked.

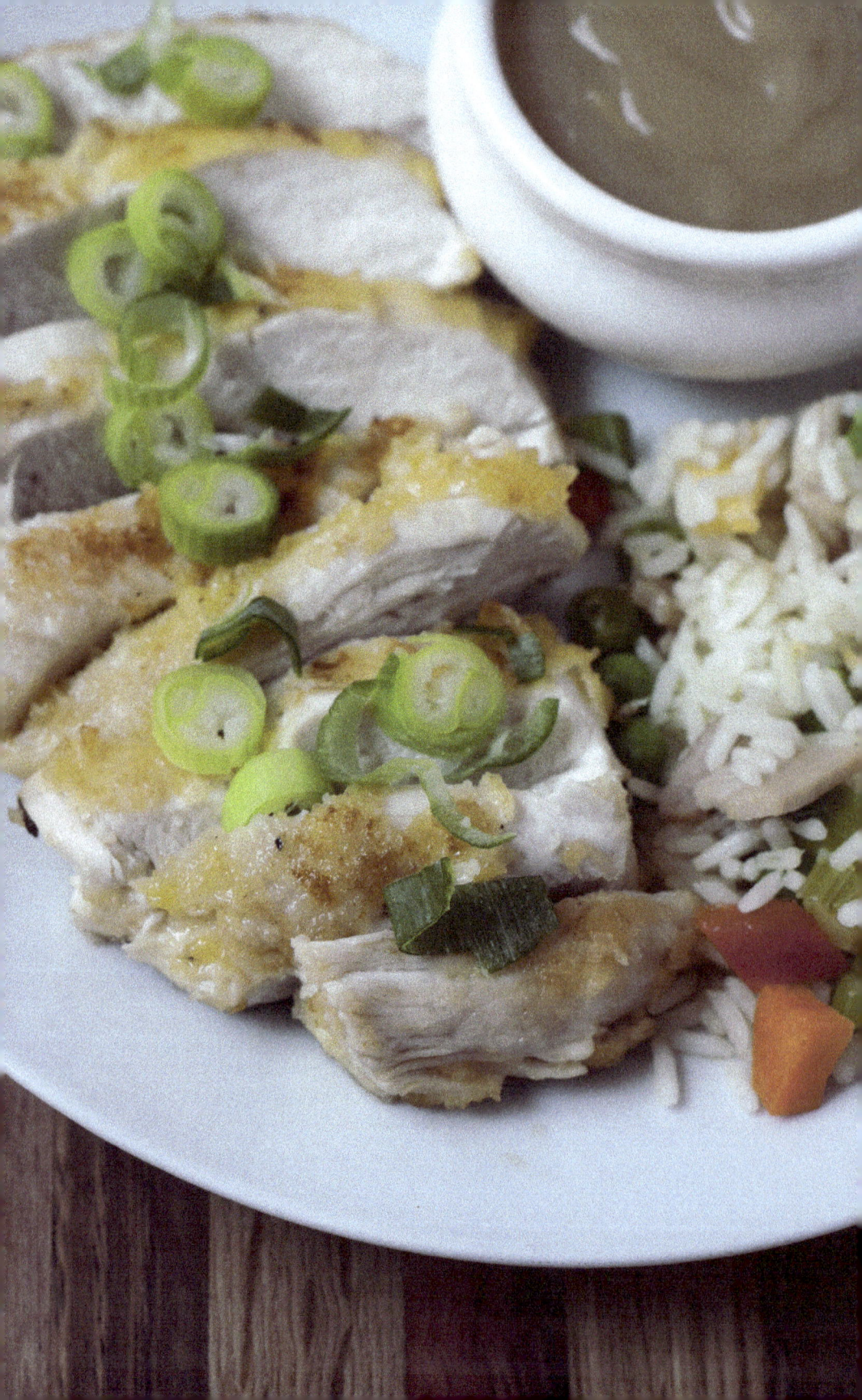

Lemon Chicken

The lemon sauce gives you both a sweet and bitter taste, but with the combination of the chicken this is a lovely, refreshing and tart dish.

INGREDIENTS
- 3 whole chicken breasts, skinned and boned
- 1/3 cup gluten-free cornflour
- 2 tablespoons water
- 6 spring onions (shallots, scallions)
- 3 egg yolks
- Oil for deep frying

Lemon Sauce:
- 2 tablespoons rice flour
- 1 ½ cups chicken stock
- 1/3 cup lemon or lime juice
- 1 teaspoon grated fresh ginger
- 1 teaspoon gluten-free soy sauce
- 1 teaspoon honey
- Sea salt, ground black pepper

METHOD
1. Cut chicken breasts in half lengthwise then pound lightly with a meat mallet.
2. Put cornflour into a bowl, gradually add water and lightly beaten egg yolks add salt and pepper and mix well.
3. Dip pieces of chicken into deep hot oil, fry in batches, until lightly golden brown and cooked through.
4. Drain on absorbent paper.
5. Keep warm until while cooking remaining chicken pieces.
6. Slice each cooked chicken breast diagonally across into three or four pieces.
7. Arrange on a plate, sprinkle with chopped shallots, spoon hot lemon sauce over the top and serve with fried rice (see page 59).

Sauce:
1. Put rice flour into a small saucepan, gradually add the chicken stock and lemon juice, stir until combined, then stir until sauce boils and thickens.
2. Add ginger, soy sauce, honey and salt and pepper.
3. Reduce heat, simmer for 3 minutes.

Serves 4.

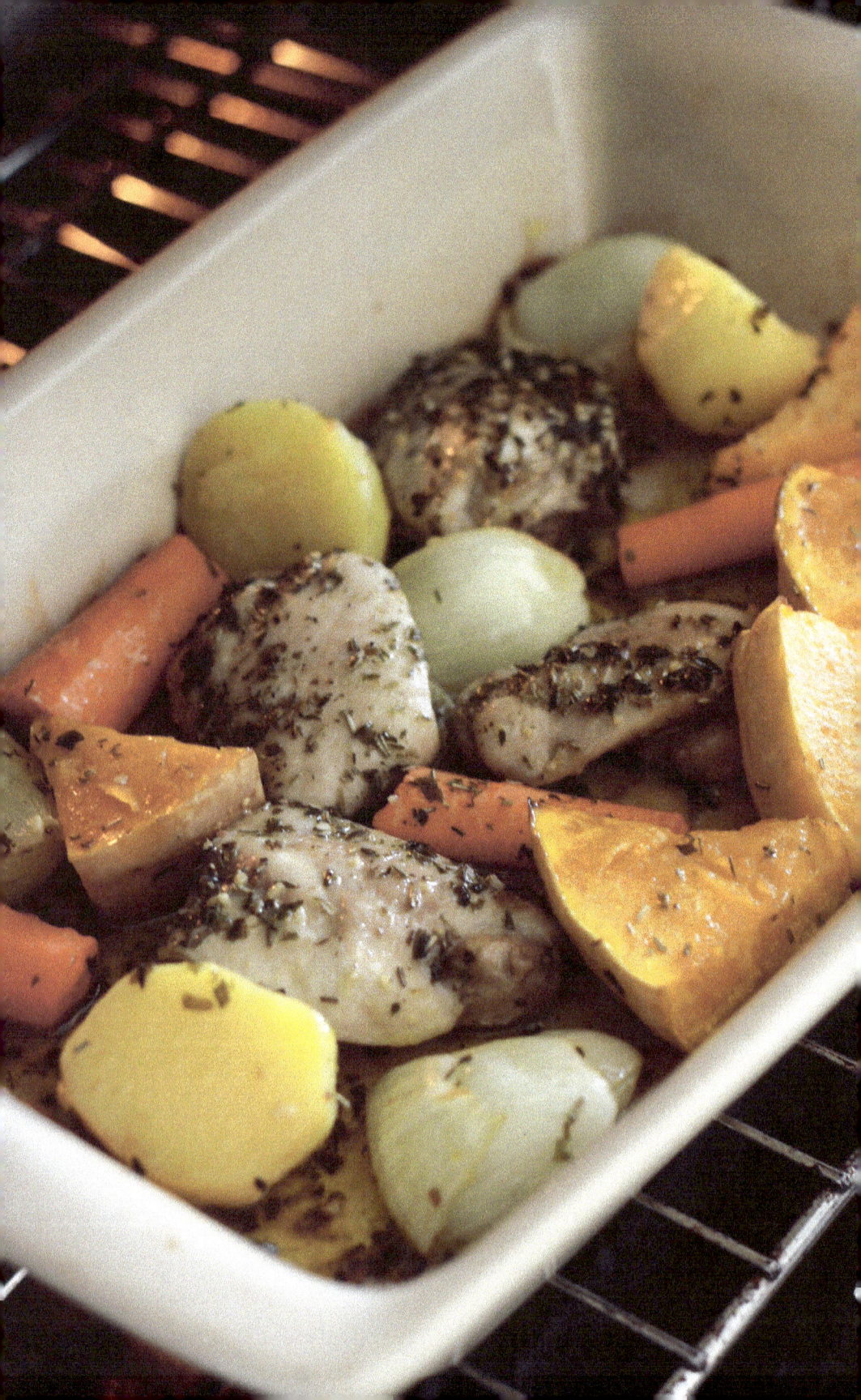

Roast Chicken

This is such an easy roast because it's all in one dish. You really just need to throw everything in and leave it! It is economical as you are using chicken thighs rather than the breast, and you can use any vegetables you enjoy with it.

INGREDIENTS
- 8 pieces organic, free range, skinned, chicken thighs (cut each piece in half)
- 2 large carrots, peeled and each carrot cut into four
- 2 large potatoes, peeled and each potato cut into four
- 4 small onions, peeled
- 4 large pieces of pumpkin
- Olive oil
- 2 teaspoons dried rosemary
- 2 teaspoons dried chives
- 2 teaspoons dried crushed garlic

METHOD
1. Heat oven to 160 degrees C (or 320 degrees F).
2. Grease a large baking dish with olive oil.
3. Place chicken and vegetable pieces into the baking dish and sprinkle with garlic, rosemary and chives.
4. Splash some more olive oil over the top of the chicken and vegetables and place the dish in the heated oven.
5. Cook for 15 to 20 minutes, turn chicken and vegetables and cook for another 15 to 20 minutes or until chicken and vegetables are cooked.

Serve with green steamed vegetables.

Serves 4.

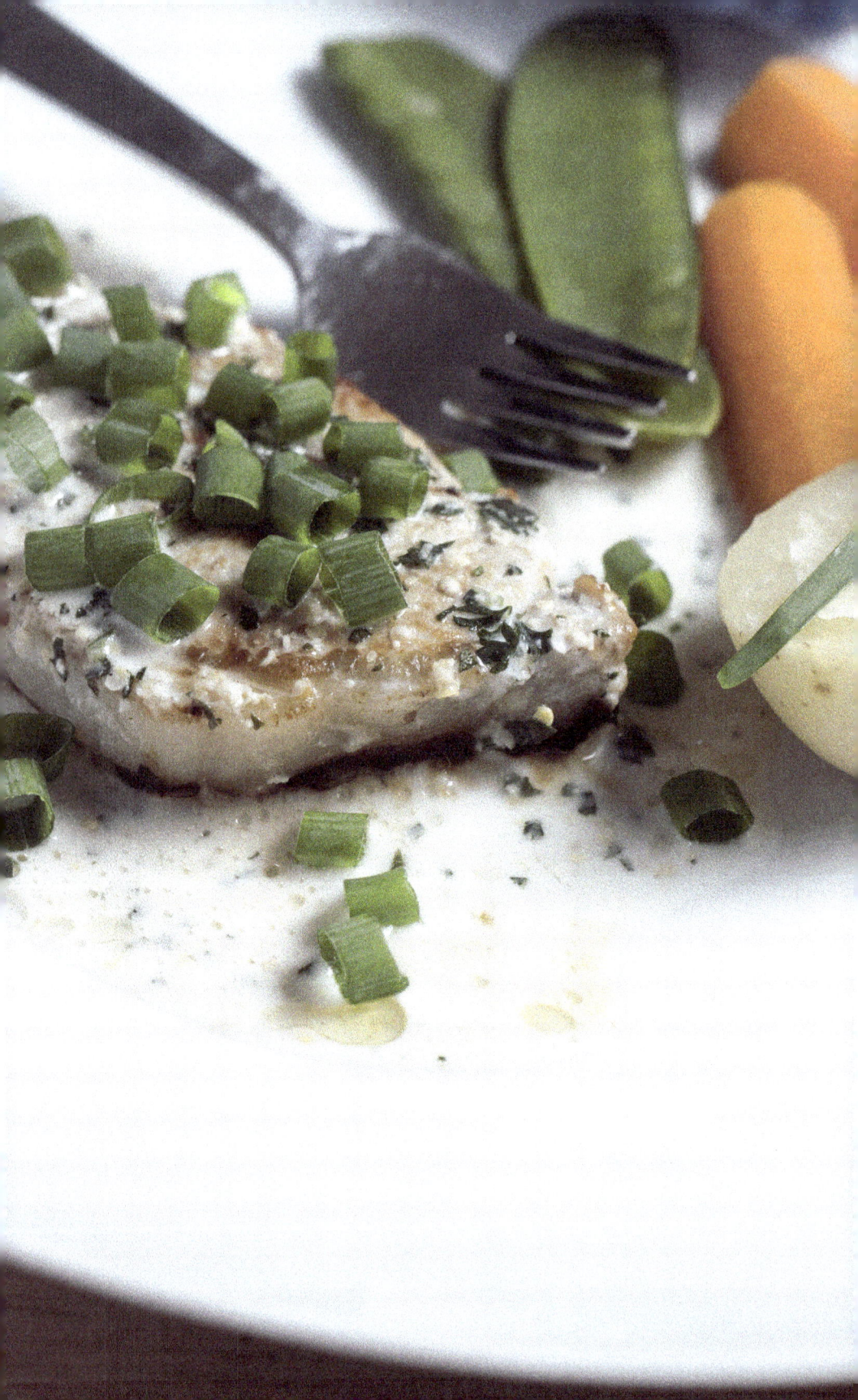

Pork With Mustard

This is a really quick and easy dish - perfect when you are in a hurry. The sauce can be premade which can make it even quicker to prepare.

INGREDIENTS
- 4 pork butterfly steaks
- 8 spring onions (shallots), finely chopped
- 2 tablespoons olive oil

METHOD
1. Heat oil in a large frying pan over high heat.
2. Brown steaks and seal.
3. Lower heat and add spring onions (shallots).
4. Continue cooking until steaks are cooked.

To serve place spring onions (shallots) on top of each steak then cover each steak with Mustard Sauce (see page 31) and add steamed vegetables of potato, carrot and snow peas.

Serves 4.

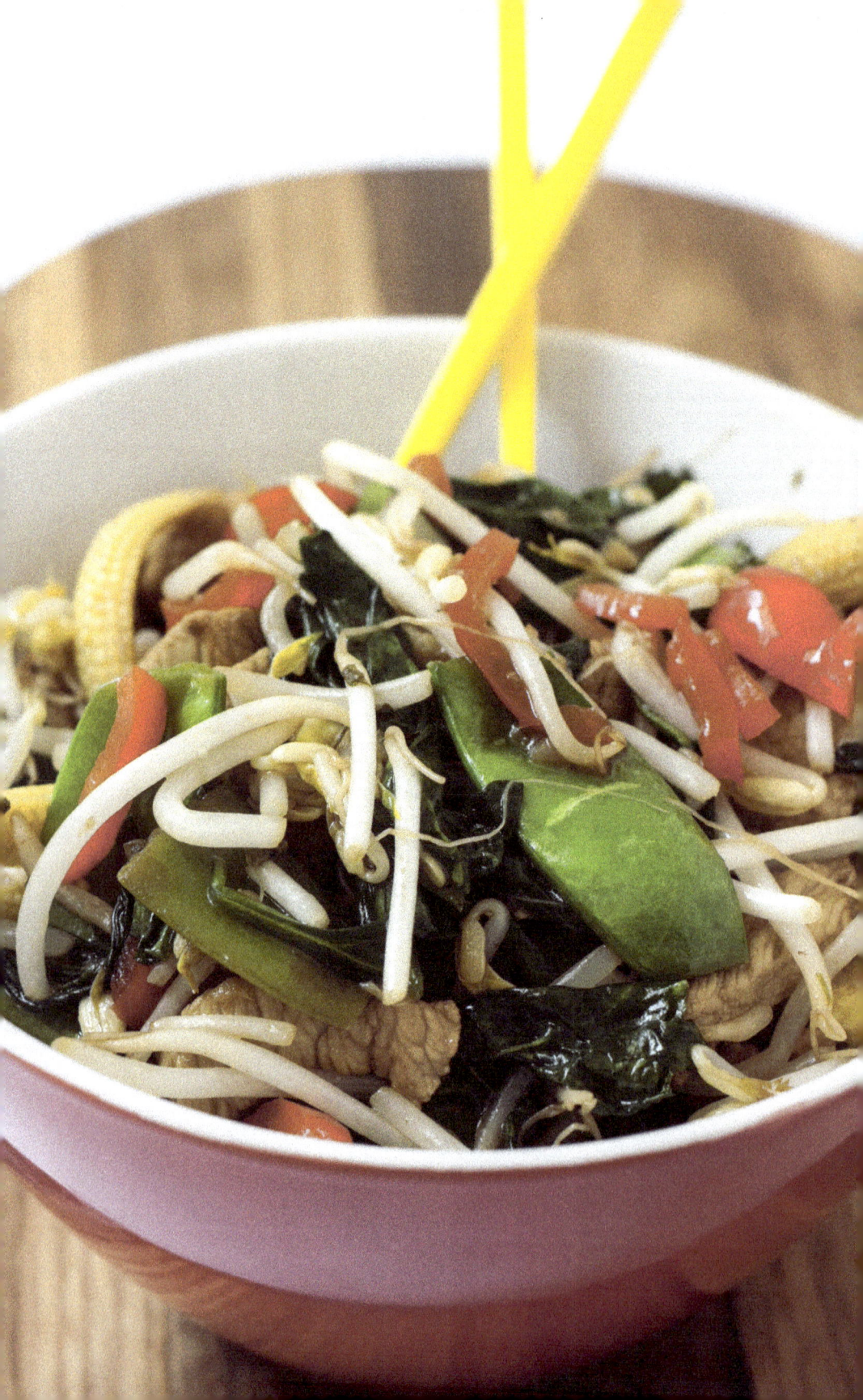

Pork Stir Fry

I really love this - the ginger flavour is wonderful and a perfect combination with the pork. Adding spinach and bean shoots makes the dish a complete meal and means that you don't require the addition of noodles or other accompaniments.

INGREDIENTS
- 700gm (1 lb 9 oz) pork fillet or steak , sliced into thin strips
- 2 tablespoons grated fresh ginger
- ¼ cup fresh coriander leaves, finely chopped
- 2 tablespoons lemon or lime juice
- 2 tablespoons of avocado or olive oil
- 120gm (4 oz) fresh baby corn , halved lengthwise
- 1 medium red capsicum (bell pepper), cut into fine strips
- 100gm (3 ½ oz) snow peas, halved
- 120gm (4 oz) spinach, trimmed
- 2 cups bean spouts
- 2 tablespoons gluten-free soy sauce
- 1 tablespoon extra coriander leaves

METHOD
1. Combine pork, ginger, coriander and juice in a medium bowl.
2. Heat half the oil in a wok or large frypan.
3. Add pork mixture in batches into the wok and stir fry until pork is brown and cooked through, remove from wok.
4. Heat remaining oil in same wok, stir fry the corn, capsicum (bell pepper) and peas until just tender, remove from wok.
5. Return pork to wok with soy sauce, stir fry until heated through.
6. Add cooked vegetables to the pork and gently toss then add spinach, sprouts and extra coriander and stir fry until spinach just wilts.

Serves 4.

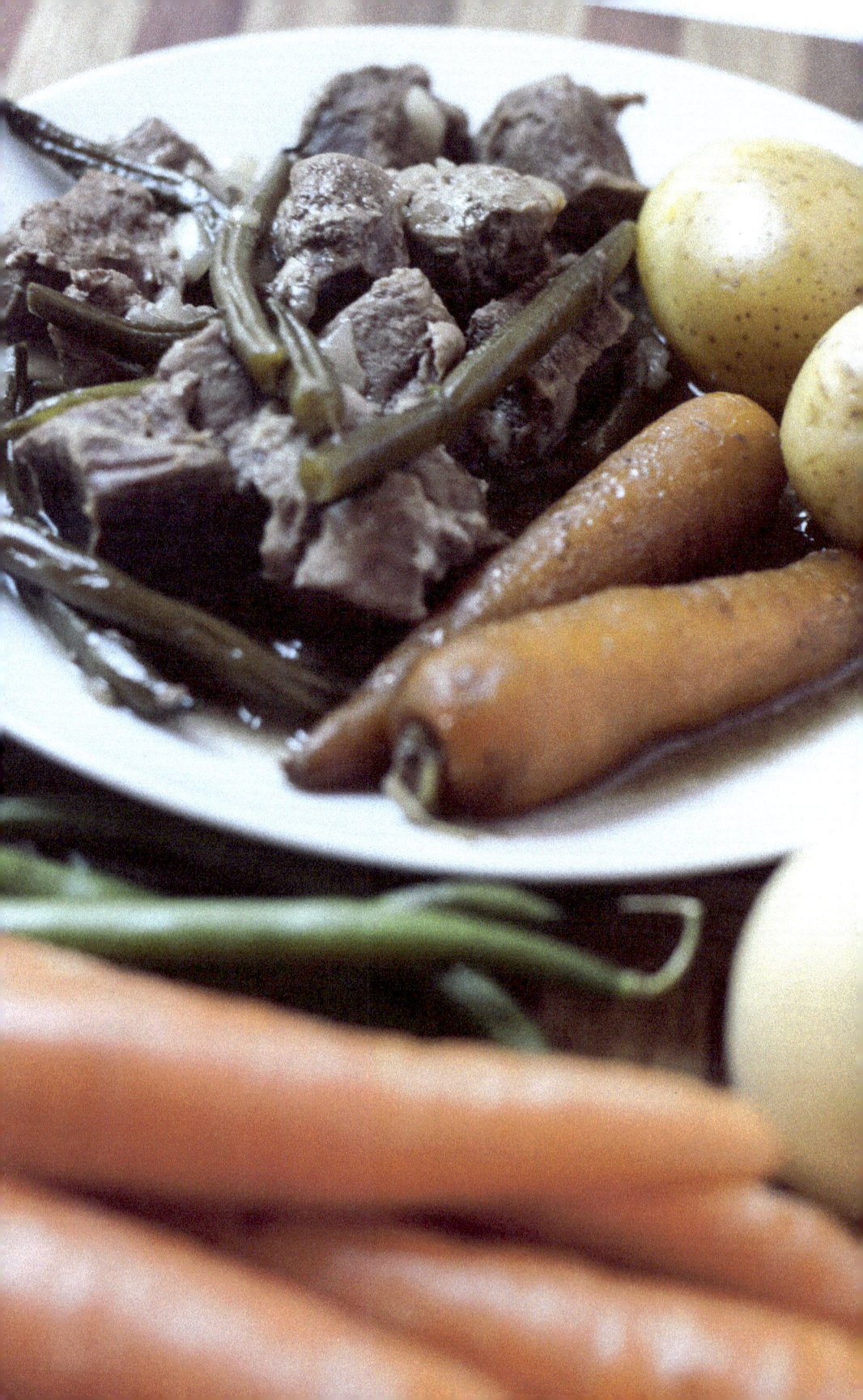

French Lamb Casserole

This is a tasty and filling recipe and it's super easy to make – just throw it all in! Just remember to take out the bouquet garni before serving or the person who bites into that will get a rude shock!

INGREDIENTS
- 500gms lean lamb cut into cubes
- 1 onion, chopped
- 1 garlic clove, crushed
- 1 tablespoon gluten-free flour
- 2 cups chicken stock (see page 35)
- Bouquet garni (see page 17)
- 8-10 chat potatoes
- 8-10 baby carrots
- Cup green beans

METHOD
1. Brown the lamb in a large pot, then remove the meat (leaving the juices).
2. Add the onion to the pot and stir until softened but brown.
3. Add the garlic and cook for another minute.
4. Return the meat to the pot and sprinkle with the flour until the meat is well coated and the liquid is starting to bubble.
5. Gradually stir in the stock. Add the bouquet garni, reduce the heat to low and simmer for 45 minutes.
6. Add the vegetables, bring to the boil and then lower to simmer for another 30 minutes. Season with salt and pepper before serving.

If you have a slow cooker, just add all the ingredients and cook on high for four hours or low for six hours – easy! Feel free to add any vegetables that are in season, the more the merrier.

Serves 5

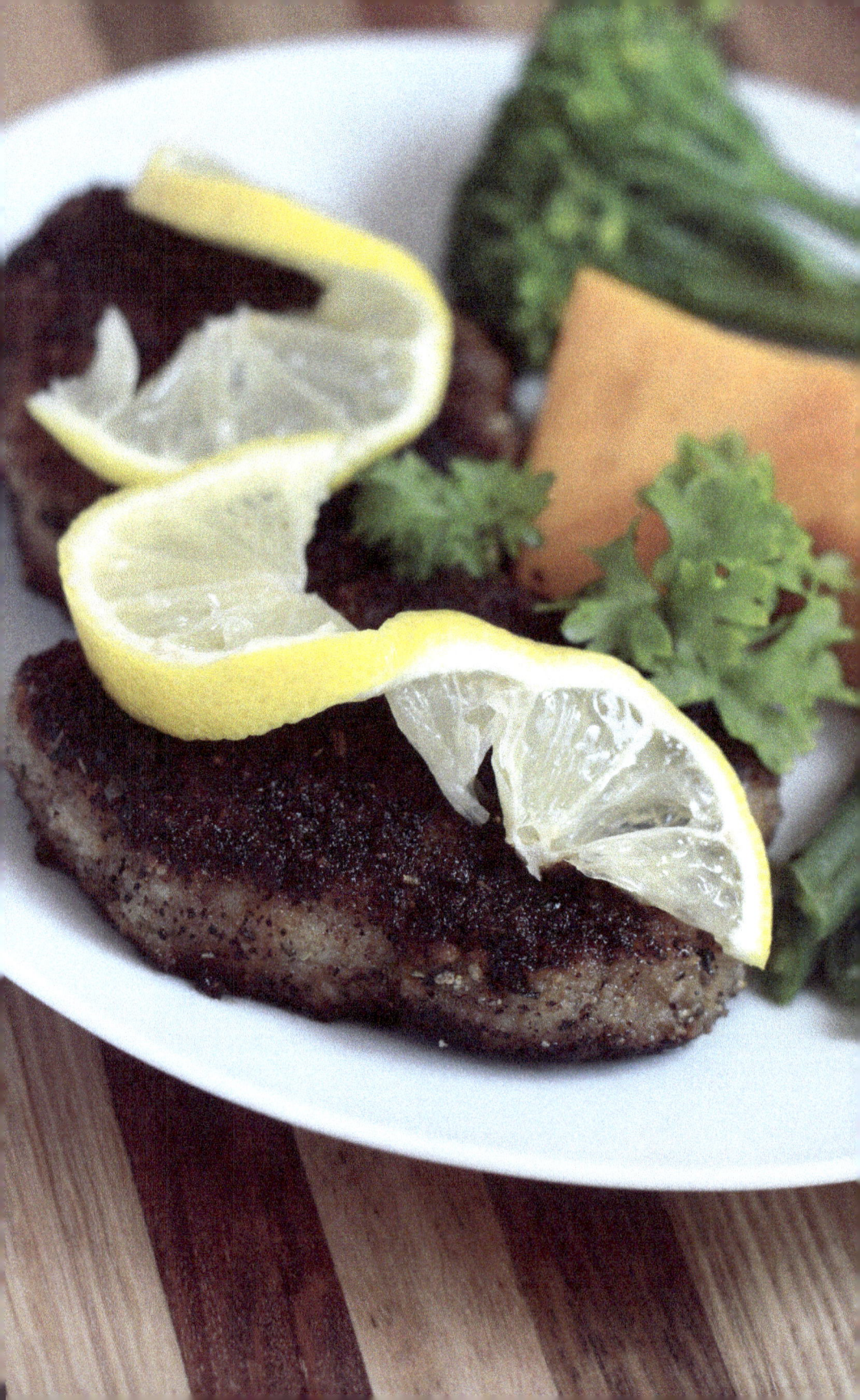

Crumbed Lamb Chops

Preservative-free and gluten-free fried food is hard to come by. This is a lovely comfort dish that still offers a little zing and a lightness with the addition of the herbs. Top it with a squeeze of fresh lemon to make it taste even lovelier.

INGREDIENTS
- 8 lamb chump chops
- 1 egg lightly beaten with 2 tablespoons water
- 1 tablespoon fresh parsley, finely chopped
- 1 tablespoon fresh chives, finely chopped
- 1 teaspoon dried thyme
- 1 teaspoon dried marjoram
- Gluten-free dried breadcrumbs
- 4 tablespoons olive oil
- Sea salt and freshly ground black pepper
- 1 Lemon or lime

METHOD
1. Trim fat and bones from lamb chops and mould into a round shape.
2. Secure with toothpicks.
3. Add herbs and salt and pepper to breadcrumbs.
4. Dip or brush chops with egg mixture and then dip each chop into the bread crumb mix, coat well – put aside in the refrigerator for 20 minutes or until ready to cook.
5. Heat oil in a heavy-based large frying pan on high heat.
6. Put lamb chops into hot oil and cook until golden brown on each side and cooked to your taste.
7. Serve topped with lemon or lime slices and steamed vegetables.

Serves 4.

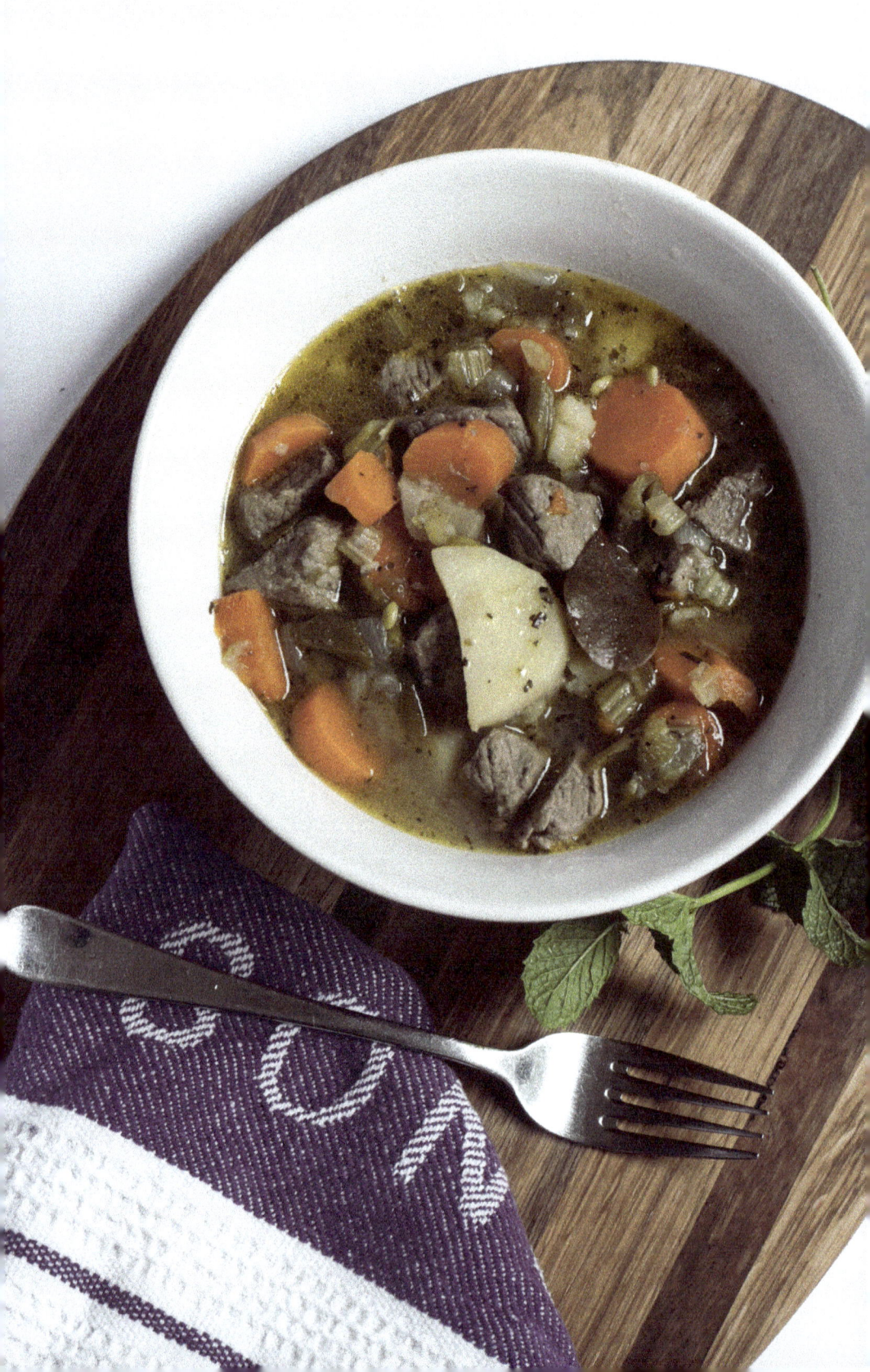

Irish Stew

This was one of the very first dishes that I modified at a time when I was really struggling because so much of my diet was restricted. When you are eating sugar-free, lamb is great because it has that little bit of sweetness - and this is also a wonderfully filling dish.

INGREDIENTS
- 500gm (1lb) lean lamb cut into 5cm (2 ½ inch) cubes
- 2 cups water
- 2 potatoes, peeled and sliced
- 2 carrots, peeled and sliced
- 1 large onion, peeled and sliced
- 1 cup chopped green beans
- 1 clove garlic, peeled and minced
- 2 bay leaves
- 1 cup sliced celery
- ½ teaspoon dried rosemary
- 1 teaspoon dried mint
- ½ teaspoon dried marjoram
- 3 tablespoons gluten-free cornflour
- 3 tablespoons olive oil
- Freshly ground black pepper and sea salt

METHOD
1. Place the cornflour in a bowl and flavour with salt and pepper, add the cut up lamb and coat in the flour.
2. Put the oil a large saucepan, put saucepan on the stove over medium heat and then add the coated lamb pieces and brown.
3. Remove the meat and add the vegetables and herbs and cook for 5 minutes.
4. Return the meat to the saucepan then slowly add the water, stirring all the time until the liquid boils and thickens.
5. Reduce the heat, cover and cook on low heat until the meat is tender to the boil. Stirring occasionally.
6. Remove bay leaves before eating.

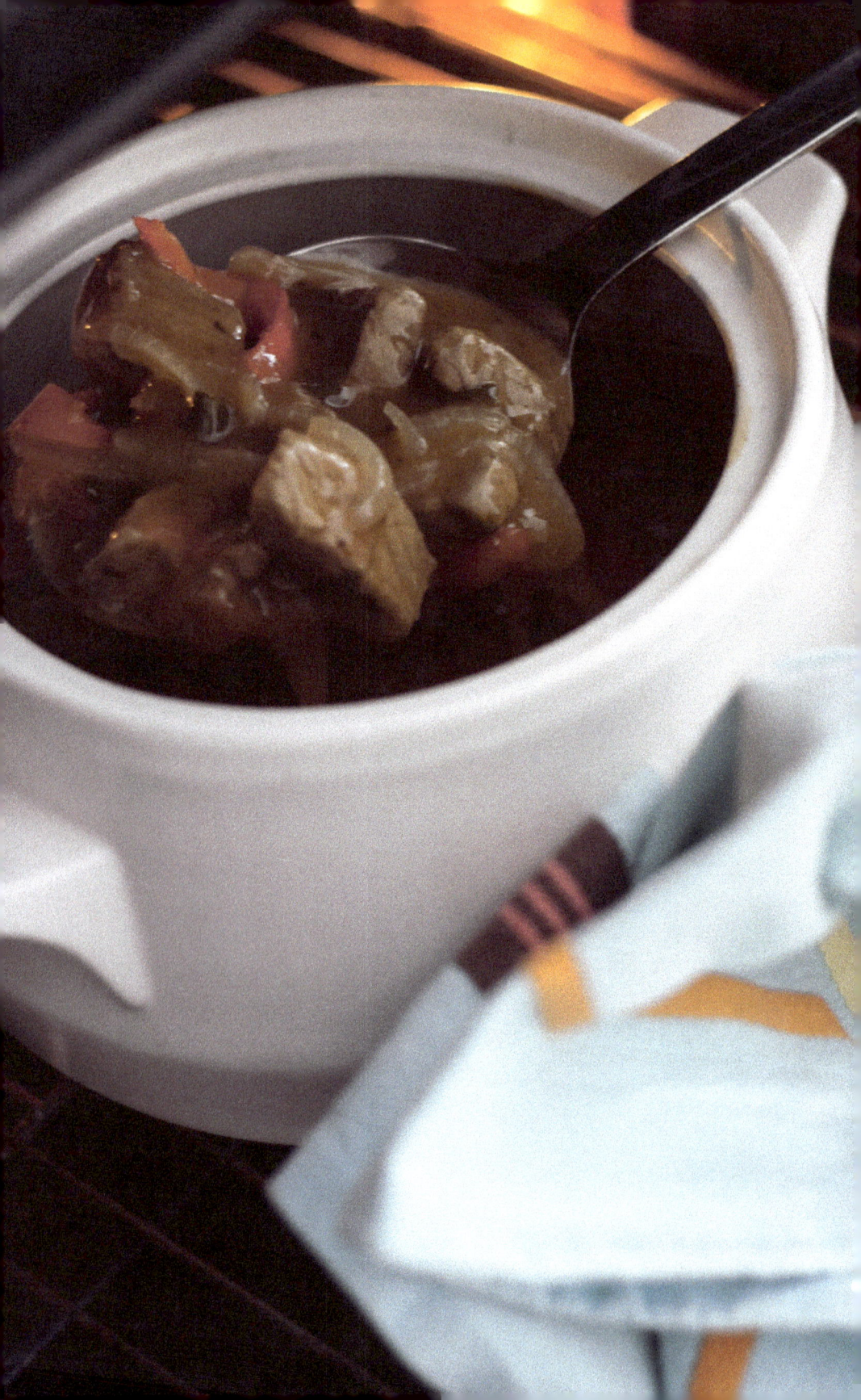

Beef Goulash

This is perfect for people who love an Eastern European flavour - it has the lovely combination of spices like paprika and marjoram that add warmth and zing to the dish. I like to serve it on mashed potato to give your palate a cooling sensation next to the spices.

INGREDIENTS
- 700gm (1lb 8oz) lean beef, cut into 5cm (2 inch)
- 3 tablespoons olive oil
- 3 tablespoons gluten-free cornflour
- ½ teaspoon sea salt
- Freshly ground black pepper
- 2 onions, peeled and cut into quarters
- 1 red capsicum (bell pepper), seeded and cut into large chunks
- 4 ripe vine tomatoes, peeled and chopped into chunks
- 2 cloves garlic, peeled and crushed
- 1 tablespoon fresh parsley, finely chopped
- ½ teaspoon dried marjoram
- 1 teaspoon hot paprika
- 1 teaspoon cumin
- 1½ cups vegetable stock (see page 37)

METHOD
1. Set oven to 160 degrees C (or 320 degrees F).
2. Combine the cornflour with salt and pepper in a dish and then add the beef cubes and coat with the seasoned flour.
3. Heat the oil in a large frypan over medium to high heat.
4. Sauté beef cubes in hot oil, in batches until well browned.
5. Put drained beef to one side.
6. Add onion pieces, cook until slightly softened, add garlic, capsicum, parsley, marjoram, paprika and cumin. Reduce heat and cook for 5 minutes.
7. Mix in tomatoes and vegetable stock and stir.
8. Put into beef pieces and vegetable mixture into a casserole dish , cover and cook in a moderate oven for 1 hour, or until the beef is tender.

Serve over mashed potatoes.

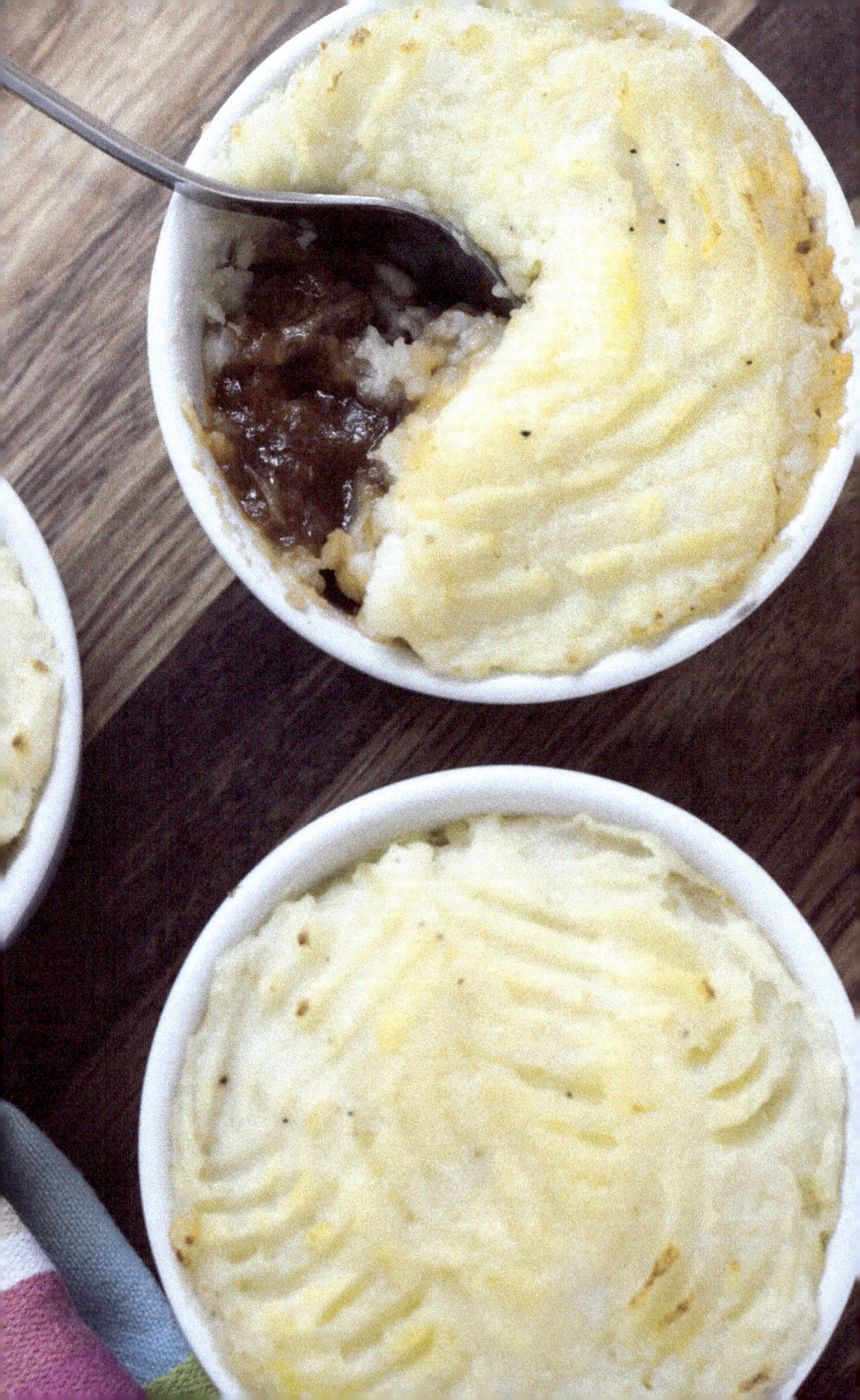

Beef Potato Pie

The original version of this (with pastry) was always a winner in our family but gluten-free, dairy-free pastry can be tricky. This version is simple, delicious and still a big hit with all family members.

INGREDIENTS
- 500 gm (1lb 2oz) rump steak, cut into small cm (¼ inch) cubes
- 1 large onion, peeled and finely chopped
- 4 thyme sprigs
- ¼ cup tomato paste
- Sea salt
- Ground black pepper
- 2 tablespoons olive oil
- ¼ cup gluten-free cornflour
- 1 ½ cups of vegetable stock (see page 37)
- 4 potatoes, peeled and quartered
- ¼ cup soy milk
- 1 tablespoon vegan spread

METHOD
1. Pre-heat oven to 180 degrees C or (350 degrees F).
2. Put the olive oil into a large frypan and heat over a medium-high heat
3. Brown the beef in 2 or 3 batches, remove each batch and put aside while the onion is cooked over low heat, remove the onions to one side.
4. Return the meat to the pan, stir in the cornflour then add the stock slowly, stirring all the time, add the cooked onions, tomato paste, and season with salt and pepper.
5. Increase the heat and keep stirring until the sauce thickens, add thyme sprigs.
6. Put the beef mixture into a casserole dish, cover the dish with a lid and place into the preheated oven and cook for 1 hour or until the beef is very tender.
7. Stir the beef every 30 minutes, making sure the beef ingredients are just covered with sauce, add more stock if necessary.
8. Whilst the beef mixture is cooking boil or steam the potatoes until tender.
9. Then mash the potatoes adding the soya milk and half the vegan spread and seasoning with salt and pepper.
10. When the beef is cooked, remove from oven and place on a heat resistant board, remove the casserole lid place to one side.
11. Remove the thyme sprigs.
12. With a large spoon divide the beef mixture into 4 individual ramekans.
13. Top each ramekan with mashed potato.
14. Spread the mashed potatoes on top of each pie with a fork dot the remaining vegan spread on top of each pie.
15. Return the pies to the oven to reheat and tops of pies are a light golden colour.

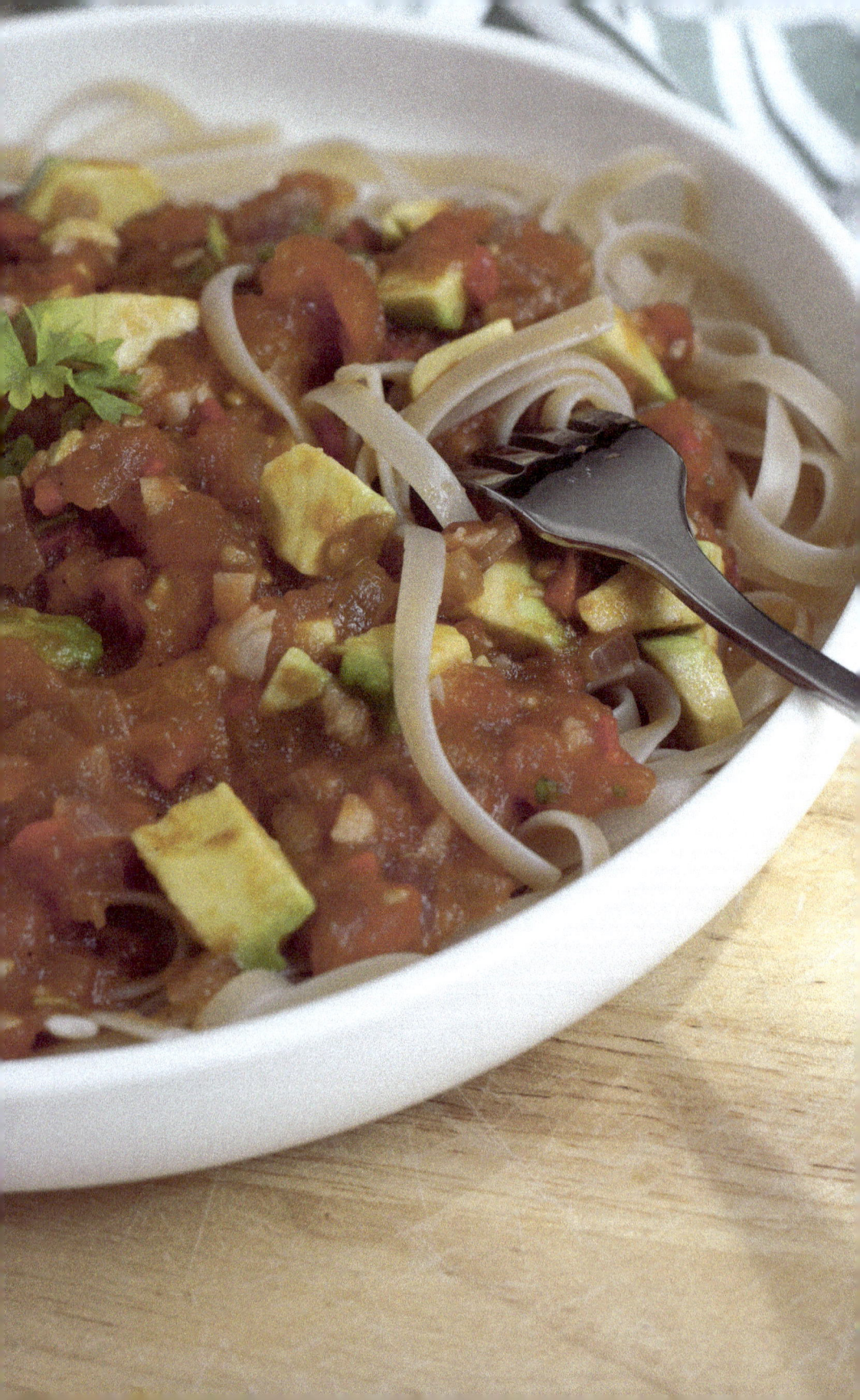

Vegetarian Pasta

Gluten-free pasta has come a long way over the years, so it's great being able to reintroduce pasta dishes to the menu. This vegetarian dish offers quite a fiery combination but the avocado helps mellow out the flavour and also offers a lovely creaminess.

INGREDIENTS
- 250gm (9oz) gluten-free fettuccine pasta
- 1 kg (2lb 4oz) vine ripened tomatoes
- 3 tablespoons olive oil
- 4 clove garlic, peeled and finely chopped
- 1 small red onion, peeled and finely chopped
- 2 bird's eye chillies, de seeded and finely chopped
- 1 ripe but firm avocado, peeled, pip removed and diced
- ½ cup fresh parsley, chopped
- Sea salt and freshly ground black pepper to taste

METHOD
Sauce:
- Cut a cross in the skin of each tomato and place in a large pot, pour boiling water over the tomatoes to cover and let stand for 3-4 minutes.
- Drain- Take the tomatoes out of the pot.
- Peel the tomatoes and discard the skin.
- Chop each tomato into small pieces.
- Heat two tablespoon of oil in a large heavy-based saucepan.
- Add the garlic and onion and cook over low heat until the onion is transparent.
- Add the tomatoes and bring to the boil then turn the heat down and simmer for 20 minutes or until the sauce has reduced and thickened.
- Add the chopped chillies into the tomato sauce and cook over low heat for another 5 minutes.
- Just before serving stir in the chopped parsley and avocado though the sauce and season with salt and cracked pepper.

Pasta:
- Fill a large saucepan with cold water and bring it to the boil.
- Add remaining 1 tablespoon of oil, then add the fettuccine.
- Cook over medium heat for 10 minutes (or according to packet instructions).
- Stir frequently so that the pasta does not stick together.
- Drain and rinse well with boiling water, then - drain again.

Serve with sauce and a mixed green salad.
Serves 4.

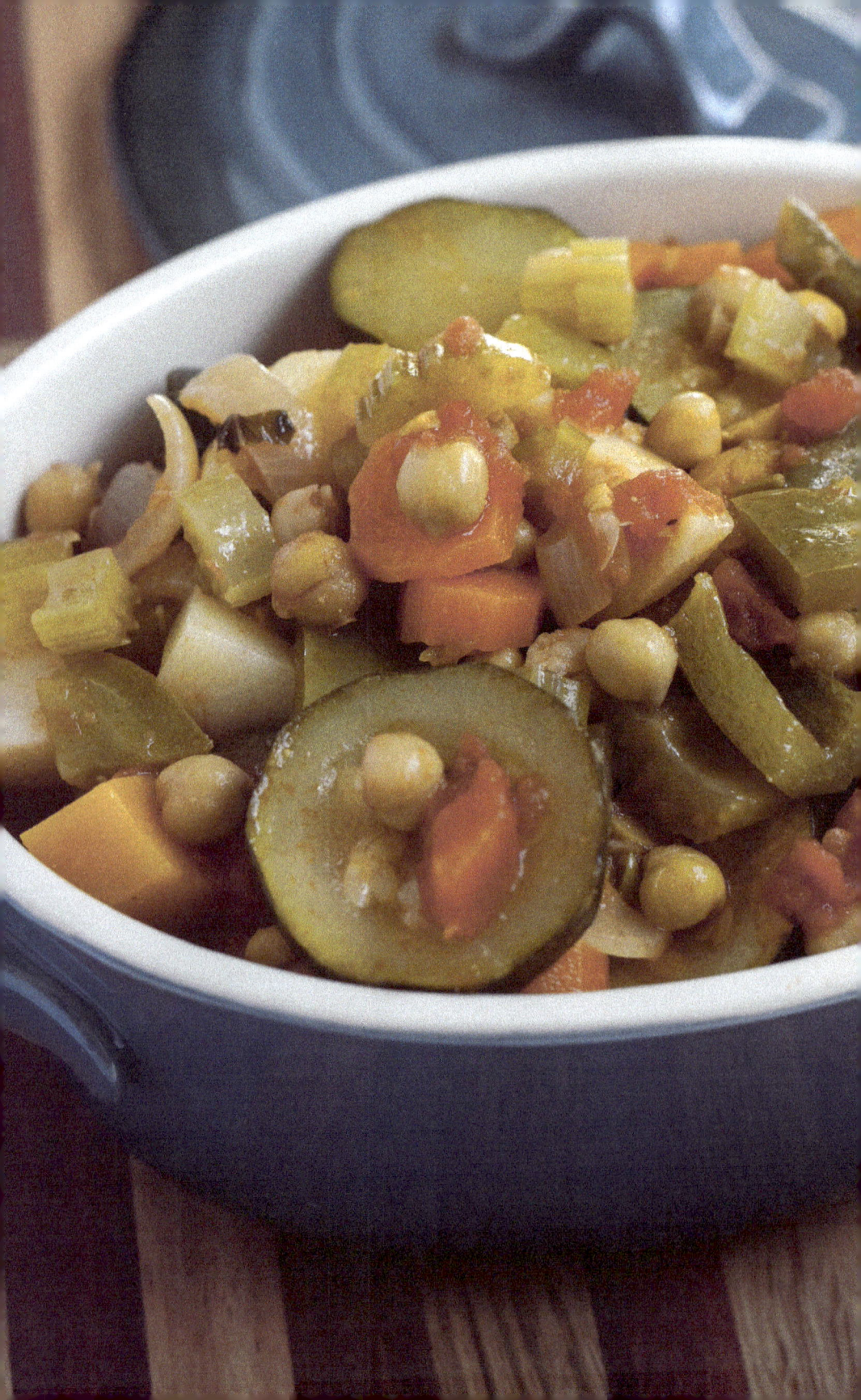

Middle Eastern Stew

This is a meal on its own, but it also makes a great side dish for any meat recipe you may enjoy. It's a great filling and healthy dish for a vegetarian - with food restrictions it can be hard to fill up at times, but it's even trickier when you don't eat meat either. This dish is perfect!

INGREDIENTS
- 1 cup vegetable stock (see page 37)
- 1 green or red capsicum (pepper), seeded and sliced
- 1 zucchini (courgette) sliced
- 200 gms (7 oz) pumpkin, seeded, peeled and cut into chunks
- 2 carrots, peeled and sliced
- 1 potato, peeled and sliced
- 1 onion, peeled, quartered and sliced
- 4 vine ripened tomatoes, peeled and chopped
- 1 birdseye chilli, deseeded and finely chopped
- 400gm (14 oz) can of beans eg chickpeas, cannellini, drained and rinsed
- 2 tablespoon chopped fresh mint
- 1 teaspoon ground cumin
- Sea salt and ground black pepper
- Extra fresh mint leaves

METHOD
1. Heat the stock in a large saucepan until boiling then add the onion, carrots, capsicum, zucchini, potato, pumpkin and celery, stir, lower heat and cook for 2-3 minutes until vegetables start to soften.
2. Add the tomatoes, chilli, mint, cumin and the beans, increase heat and bring to the boil, then reduce heat again, cover and simmer for 30 minutes or until vegetables are tender.
3. Season with salt and pepper to taste and garnish with mint leaves.

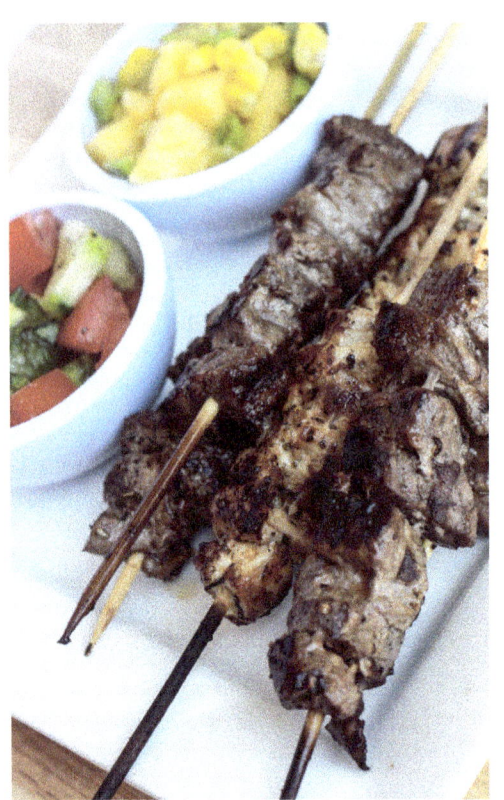
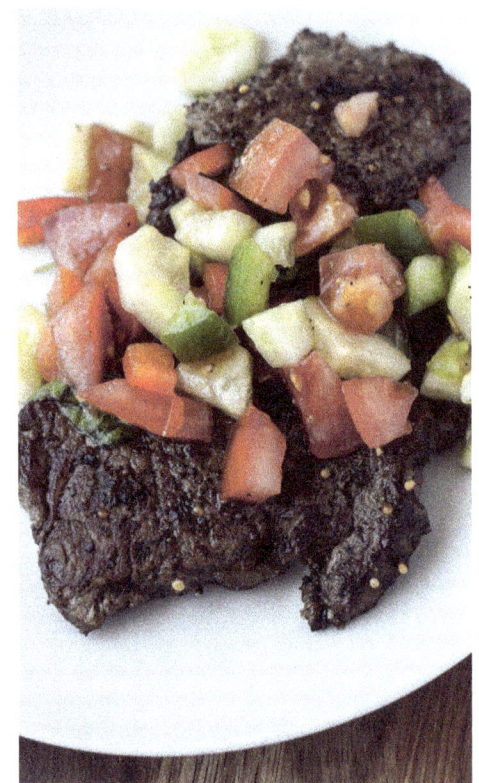
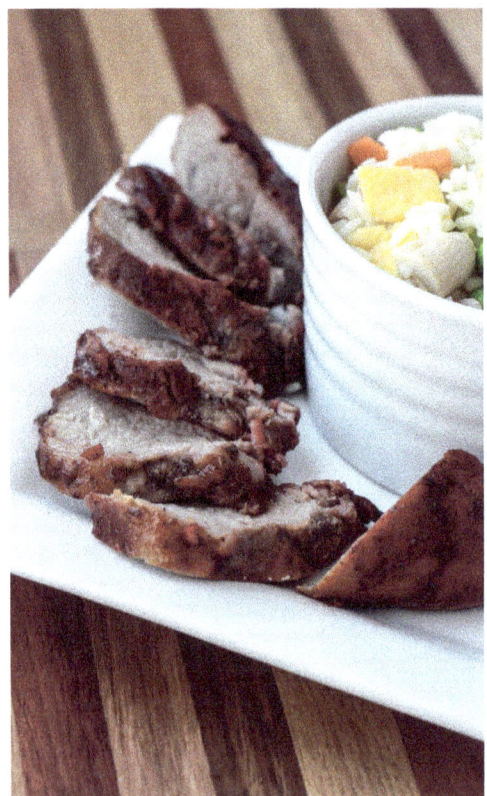
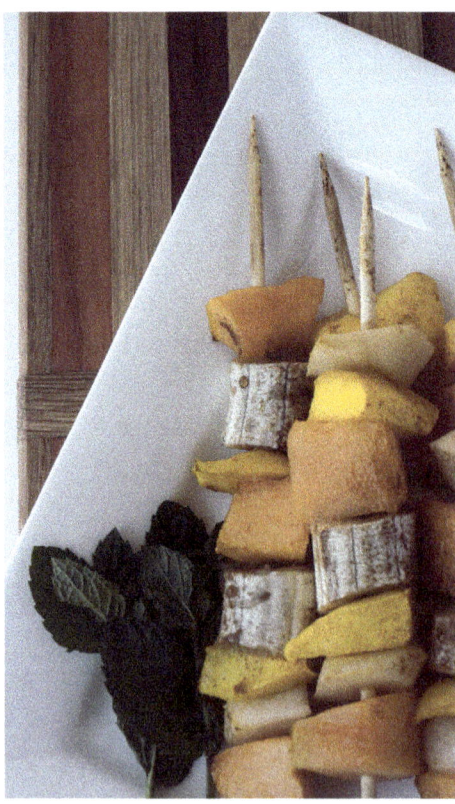

BBQ

BBQs are a social, inclusive way to socialise...and often a nightmare for people with food allergies or food intolerances! Here are some fabulous recipes for everyone to enjoy (just be sure to use a Teflon sheet or hotplate liner if you're sharing a BBQ hot plate with other food that may not be so allergy-friendly).

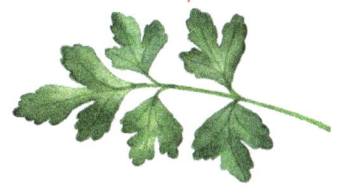

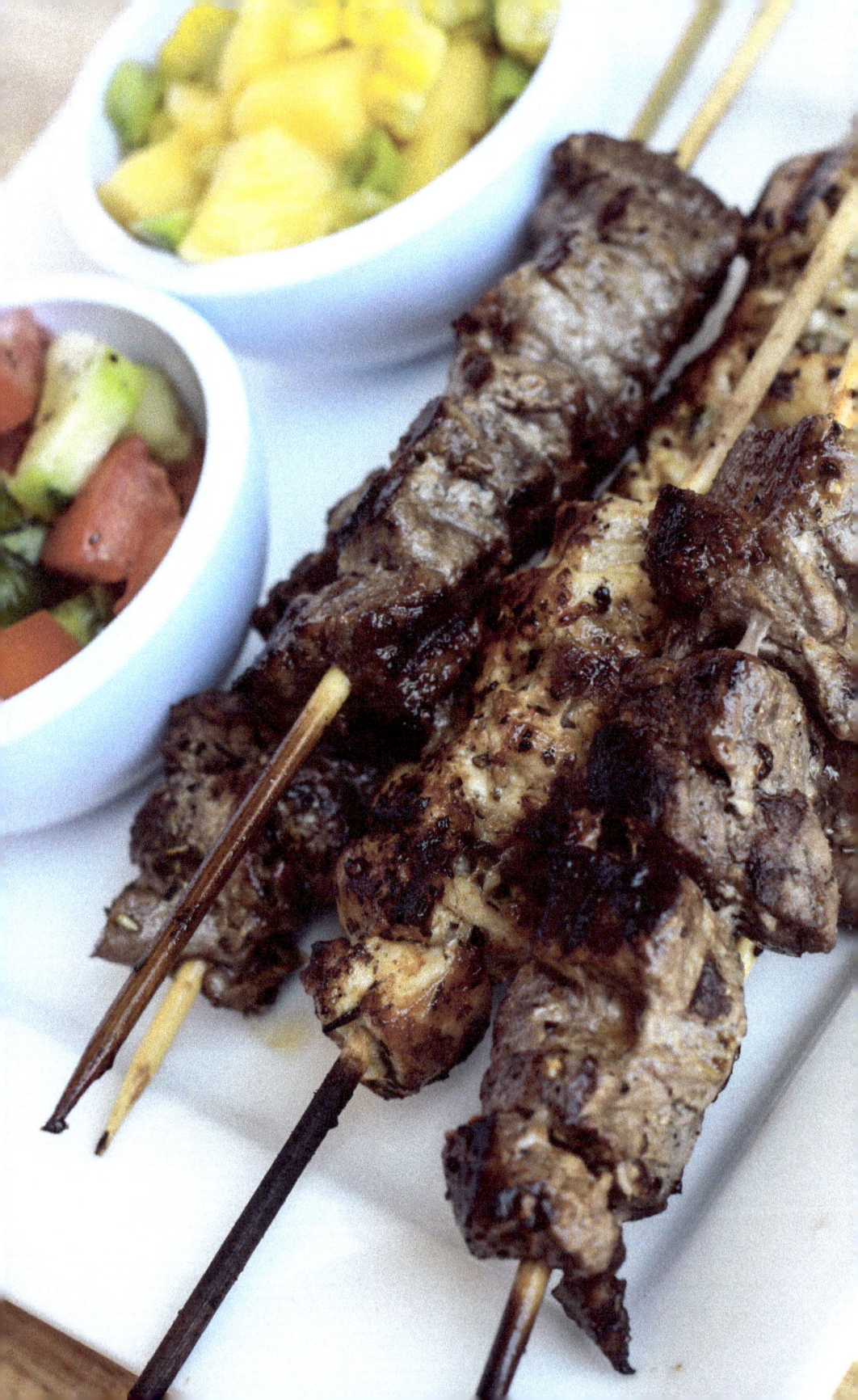

Chicken Kebabs

This marinade is very popular with children - despite the use of paprika and cumin. it isn't too spicy and still offers plenty of flavour. Chicken is always a family favourite as well!

INGREDIENTS
- 500gm (1 lb) free range organic chicken breasts, cut in half and then into 2.5cm (1 inch) cubes

Marinade:
- 2 tablespoons basil and tomato herbed oil (see page 27)
- 2 teaspoons paprika
- 1 teaspoon ground cumin
- 2 cloves garlic, peeled and crushed
- 1 tablespoon fresh oregano

METHOD
1. Combine all the marinade ingredients into a large shallow ceramic dish.
2. Add the diced chicken, cover with cling wrap and refrigerate overnight. Turning occasionally.
3. Soak long bamboo skewers in water for at least 2 hours, to prevent skewers burning on the barbecue.
4. Remove chicken cubes from the marinate and thread evenly onto the skewer sticks.
5. Cook on a heated barbecue plate or grill for 5 minutes on each side.

Lamb Kebabs

The mint and rosemary flavour creates a lovely fresh and sweet taste... and a lamb lover will adore these kebabs!

INGREDIENTS
- 500gm (1 lb) lamb cut into 2.5cm (1 inch) cubes

Marinade:
- 2 tablespoons virgin olive oil
- 1 clove garlic, peeled and crushed
- 2 teaspoons finely grated lemon or lime rind
- 4 sprigs of fresh rosemary
- 1 tablespoon finely chopped fresh mint
- 1 tablespoon finely chopped fresh majoram
- 1 tablespoon finely chopped fresh parsley
- Freshly ground black pepper and sea salt to flavour

METHOD
1. Place lamb cubes in a ceramic dish.
2. Mix marinade ingredients in a bowl and stir through.
3. Pour marinade over lamb cubes, cover with cling wrap.
4. Refrigerate over night.
5. Soak bamboo skewers in water over night to stop them burning on the barbecue.
6. Thread the drained beef evenly onto the skewers.
7. Cook on the barbecue grill for 5 minutes on each side.

Beef Kebabs

Beef, capsicum and coriander are all very masculine flavours that the boys seem to love. To give it a little edge, the ginger in this recipe creates an extra tang and freshness that is perfect for warm days.

INGREDIENTS
- 500gm (1 lb) rump steak, cut into 2.5cm (1 inch) cubes

Marinade:
- ¼ cup garlic oil (page 25)
- 1 clove garlic, peeled and crushed
- 1 tablespoon lemon or lime juice
- 1 teaspoon grated fresh ginger
- 1 tablespoon red capsicum (pepper), seeded and finely diced
- ½ teaspoon ground coriander
- Freshly ground black pepper and sea salt to season

METHOD
1. Place cubed steak in ceramic dish.
2. Combine marinade ingredients together in a bowl.
3. Pour marinade over steak pieces, cover dish with cling wrap and refrigerate over night.
4. Soak bamboo skewers in water for a few hours or over night so they won't burn on the barbecue.
4. Thread steak pieces evenly onto bamboo skewers.
5. Place skewers onto barbecue grill and for 5 minutes on each side.

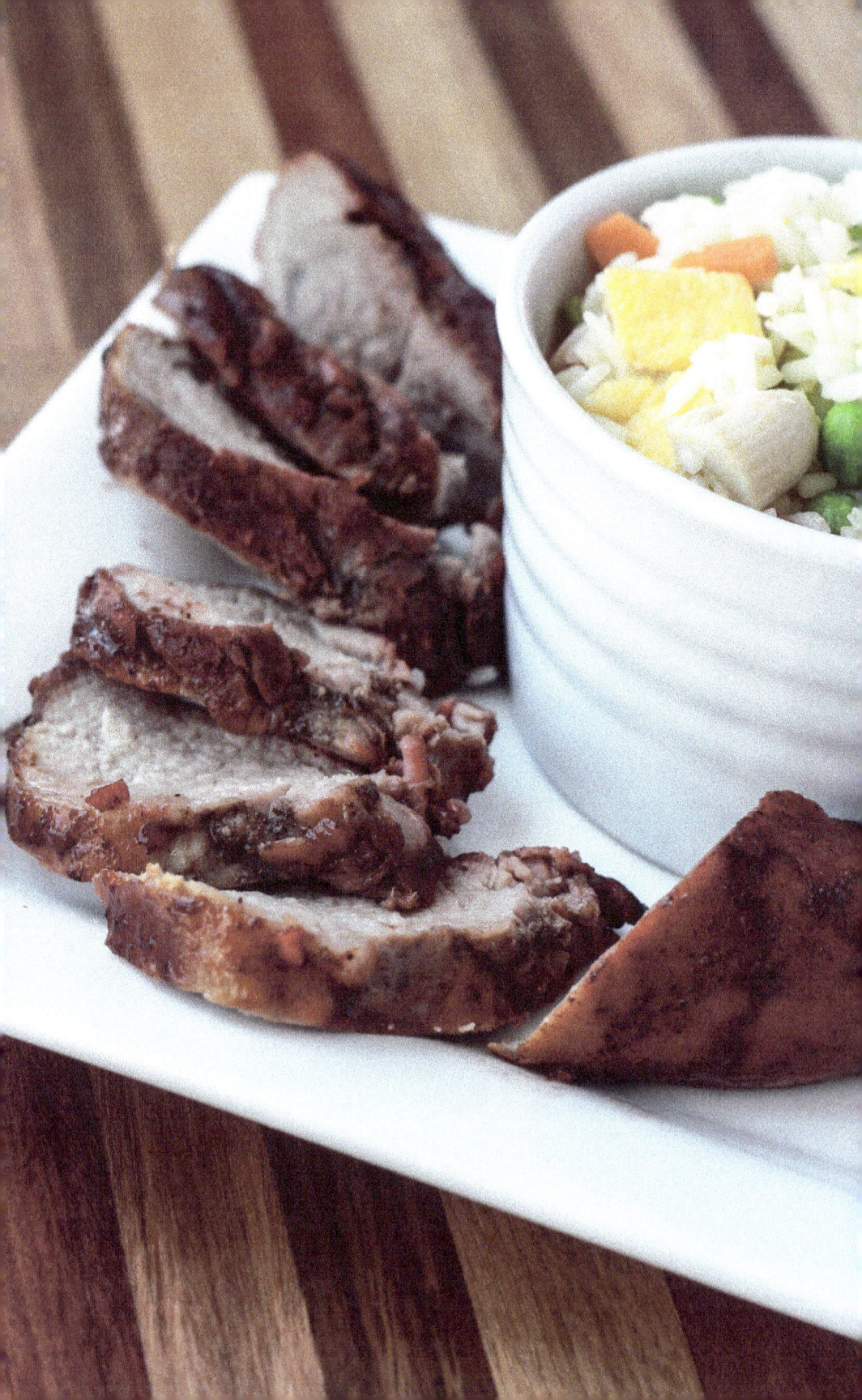

Asian-style Pork

When my children were little, I liked to create meals from other countries. We often had a 'Chinese' night and this was a favourite. The red food colouring meant that this dish was off the menu for me with my new diet, but using beetroot as a substitute, I have found a way to recreate it (and I think this version is actually even better!)

INGREDIENTS
- 2 lean pork fillets
- ¼ cup gluten-free soy sauce
- 2 tablespoons lemon or lime juice
- 1 tablespoon honey
- 1 clove garlic crushed
- 1 spring onion (shallot or scallion)
- ½ teaspoon cinnamon
- 2 small fresh beetroots, cooked, peeled and sliced
- 3 tablespoons beetroot water

METHOD
1. Pre-heat oven to 160 degrees C (or 350 degrees F).
2. Place two beetroots in a small saucepan, cover with water, bring to the boil on high heat, reduce heat and cook beetroot until it is tender.
3. Mix gluten free soy sauce, juice, honey, garlic, halved shallot and beetroot water together in a large ceramic bowl.
4. Sprinkle cinnamon on top, add pork and sliced beetroot.
5. Cover the dish with cling wrap and place in the refrigerator and marinate for at least one hour or overnight, turning the pork leans occasionally.
6. Drain the pork fillets from the marinade, reserving the marinade.
7. Put pork fillets on a wire rack over a baking dish or on a BBQ grill.
8. Bake in a moderate oven for 30-40 minutes, turning frequently with tongs and basting often with reserved marinade. If grilling on the BBQ, still top with the marinade and allow 15-20 minutes turning frequently.
9. Remove from the oven (or grill), put onto a board and allow to cool slightly.
10. Cut pork into diagonal slices to serve.

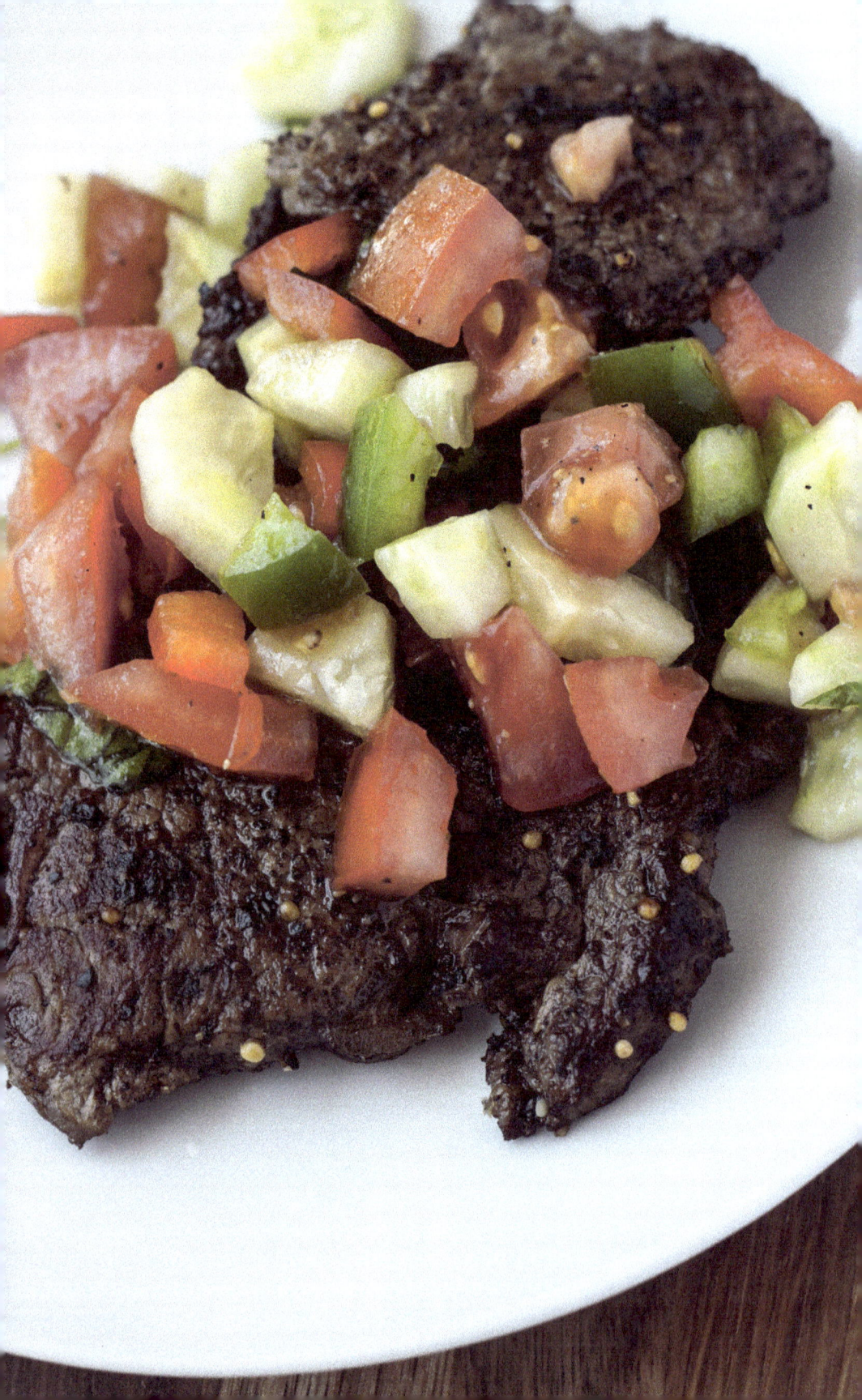

Peppered Steaks

The men in my family all love this dish - a great version of the traditional steak with pepper sauce. It is simple to prepare and great when cooked on the BBQ. The mustard really adds that extra flavour.

INGREDIENTS
- 4 beef fillet steaks
- 2 tablespoons black peppercorns
- 1 tablespoon white mustard seeds
- 2 tablespoon of garlic oil (see page 25)

METHOD
1. Trim any excess fat off the steaks.
2. Put the steaks between two sheets of plastic wrap and flatten the steaks with a meat mallet.
3. Nick the edges of the steak to prevent the steak from curling when cooking.
4. Crush the peppercorns and mustard seeds until coarsely crushed.
5. Rub oil over the steak, then press on the peppercorn mixture to coat both sides.
6. Store in the refrigerator covered in new plastic wrap for 30 minutes.
7. Cook the steak on a hot, lightly oiled barbecue flatplate or grill for 2 minutes on each side.
8. For rare steaks cook for a further 1 minute on each side.
8. For medium to well done steaks, move the steaks to a cooler part of the barbecue and cook for a further 3-6 minutes on each side.

Serves 4.

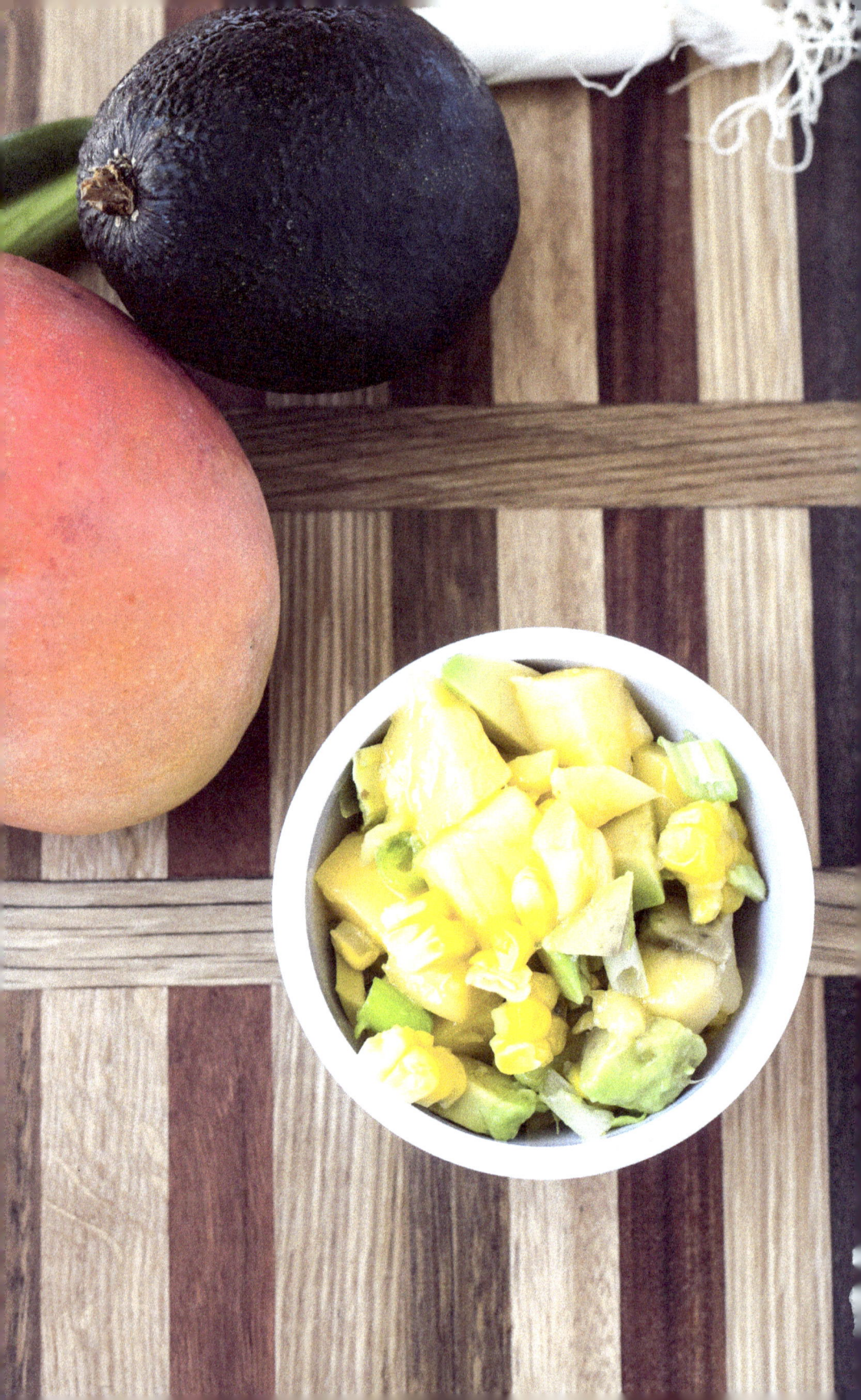

Mango Salsa

This is one of my favourites - I love the sweetness that it gives and it is a perfect match with chicken or pork. It is also has a lovely creamy texture that is very filling. It can also make a great pre-BBQ snack with crackers.

INGREDIENTS
- 1 large ripe mango, peeled, stoned and chopped
- 1 large ripe avocado, peeled, stoned and chopped
- 1 cooked corn on the cob
- 1 spring onion (shallot), finely chopped
- 1 tablespoon lime juice

METHOD
1. Mix all ingredients together.
2. Leave salsa in the refrigerator until ready to use.

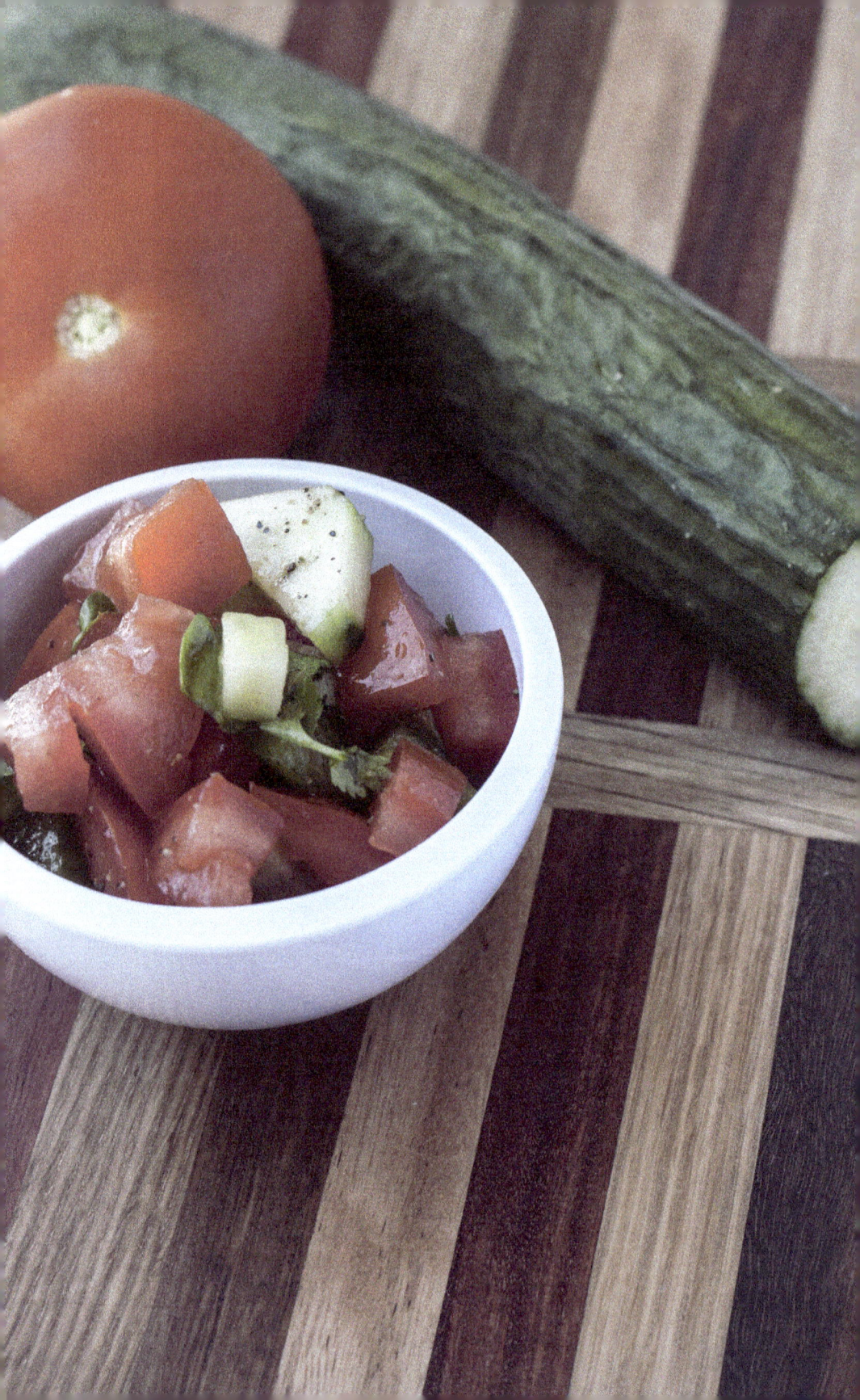

Tomato Salsa

This salsa is lovely, refreshing and absolutely delicious to enjoy on any grilled or fried meat. On its own it can be a great light summer appetiser.

INGREDIENTS
- 1 small cucumber, peeled and diced
- 1 red tomato, diced
- 1 small red onion, peeled and diced
- 2 tablespoons Basil and Sundried Tomato Oil (See Page 27)
- 1 tablespoon lemon or lime juice
- 1 tablespoon fresh coriander, chopped
- 1 tablespoon fresh basil, chopped

METHOD
1. Mix all ingredients together.
2. Leave salsa in the refrigerator until ready to use.

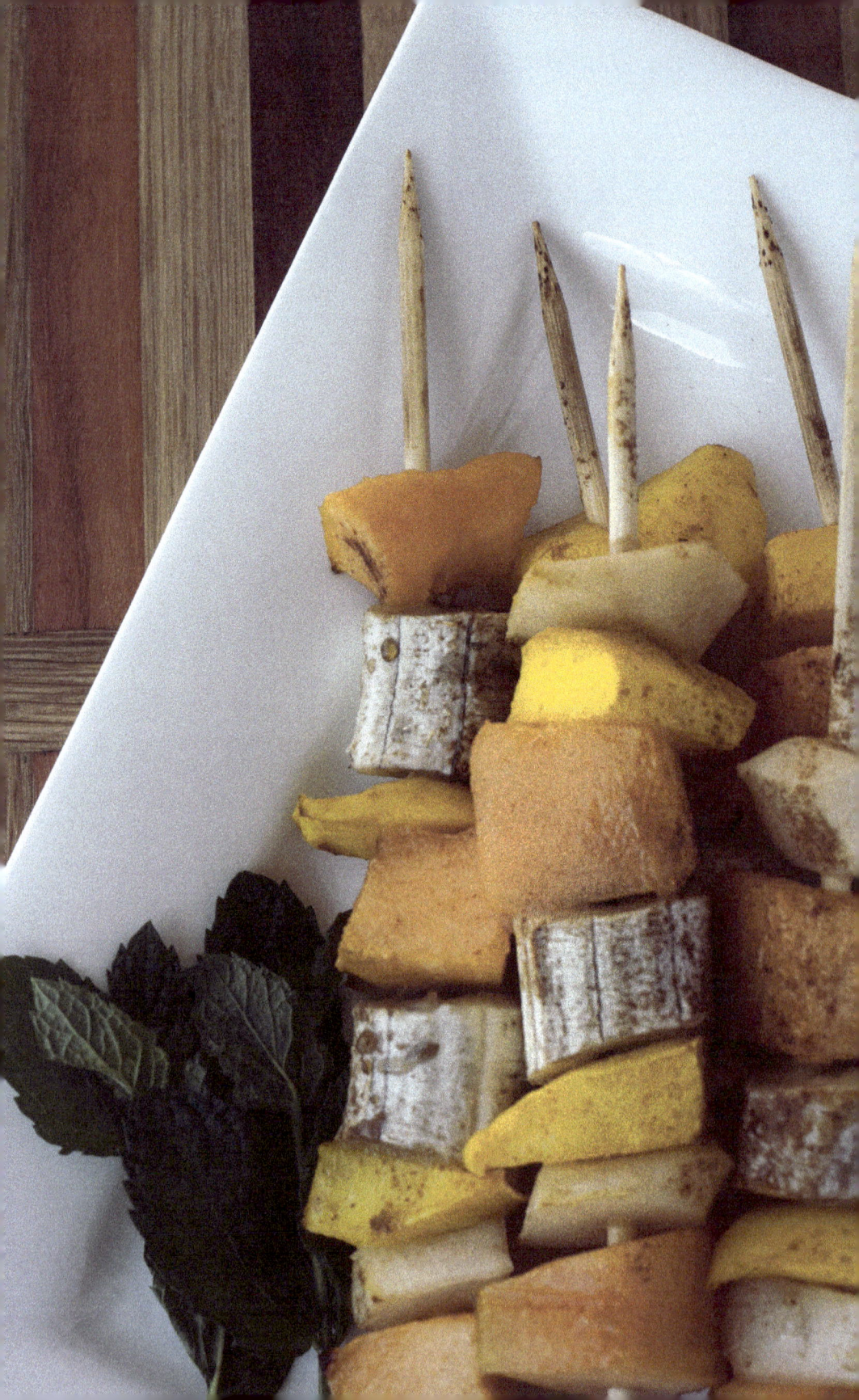

Fruit Kebabs

These can be served cold, although cooking them on a BBQ offers a unique and delicious flavour. You can use pretty much any fruit that is in season - so definitely feel free to experiment!

INGREDIENTS
- 1 ripe firm mango, peeled and cut into chunks
- ½ cantaloupe (rockmelon), peeled, seeded and cut into chunks
- 4 ripe firm pears, peeled, cored and cut into chunks
- 4 ripe firm bananas, peeled and cut into chunks
- Lemon or lime juice
- 4 tablespoons of pure maple syrup
- Ground nutmeg
- Sunflower oil

METHOD
1. Soak 4 bamboo skewers in water for 2 hours (to stop burning on the barbecue or grill).
2. Place the cut pears and bananas in the lemon or lime juice to stop the fruit browning.
3. Evenly thread the fruit onto the skewer, with a piece of mango, pear, cantaloupe and banana.
4. Cut a piece of foil the length of the kebabs that is wide enough to hold the four (or however many you are making) plus a little extra to roll up an edge (so it is like a foil plate!)
5. Lightly grease the foil with oil, then lay the kebabs onto the foil, drizzle with maple syrup and sprinkle some nutmeg on top.
6. Place on the grill and gently cook for 5 minutes.

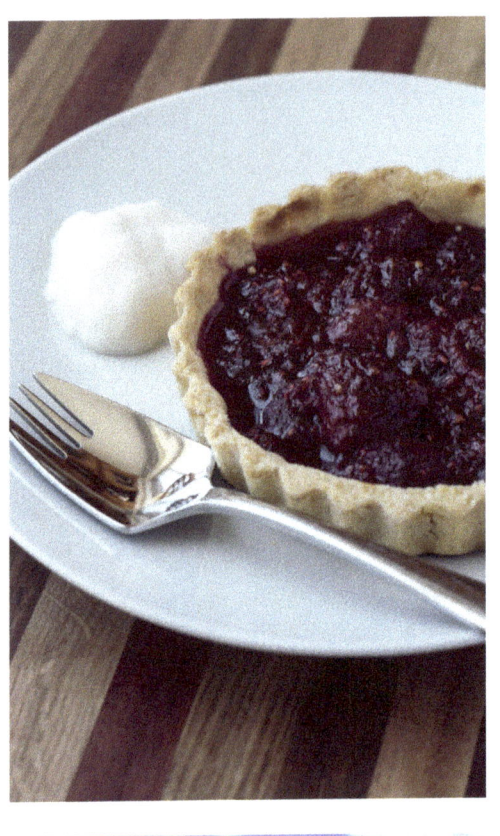
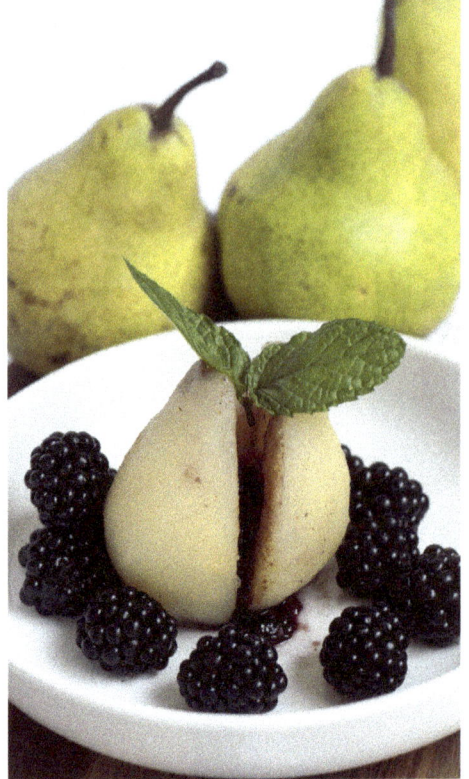
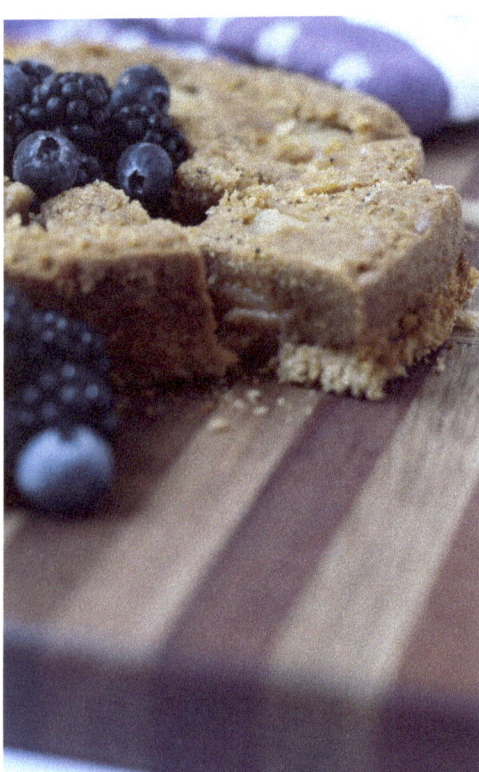
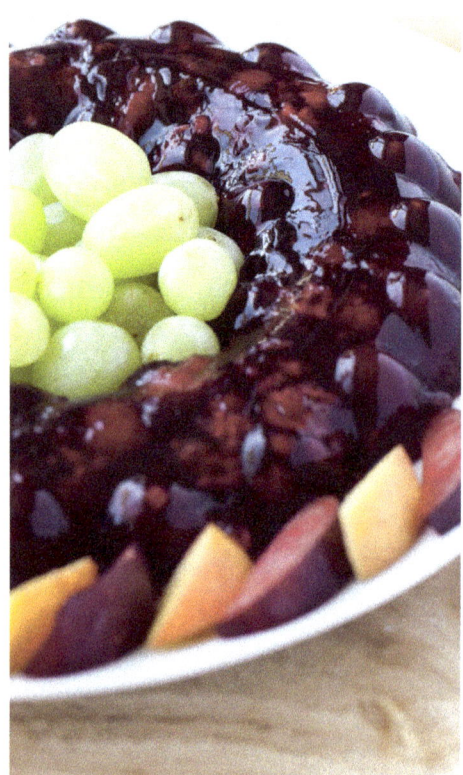

DESSERTS

On the whole, I try to avoid dessert as too much sweetness can bring on a migraine. However, for special occasions, I look to low GI options. Refined sugar can cause havoc with your immune system and it's immediately addictive, so look at options such as rice syrup to make life easier. The trick with dessert is to eat it in moderation...and share everything with friends and family!

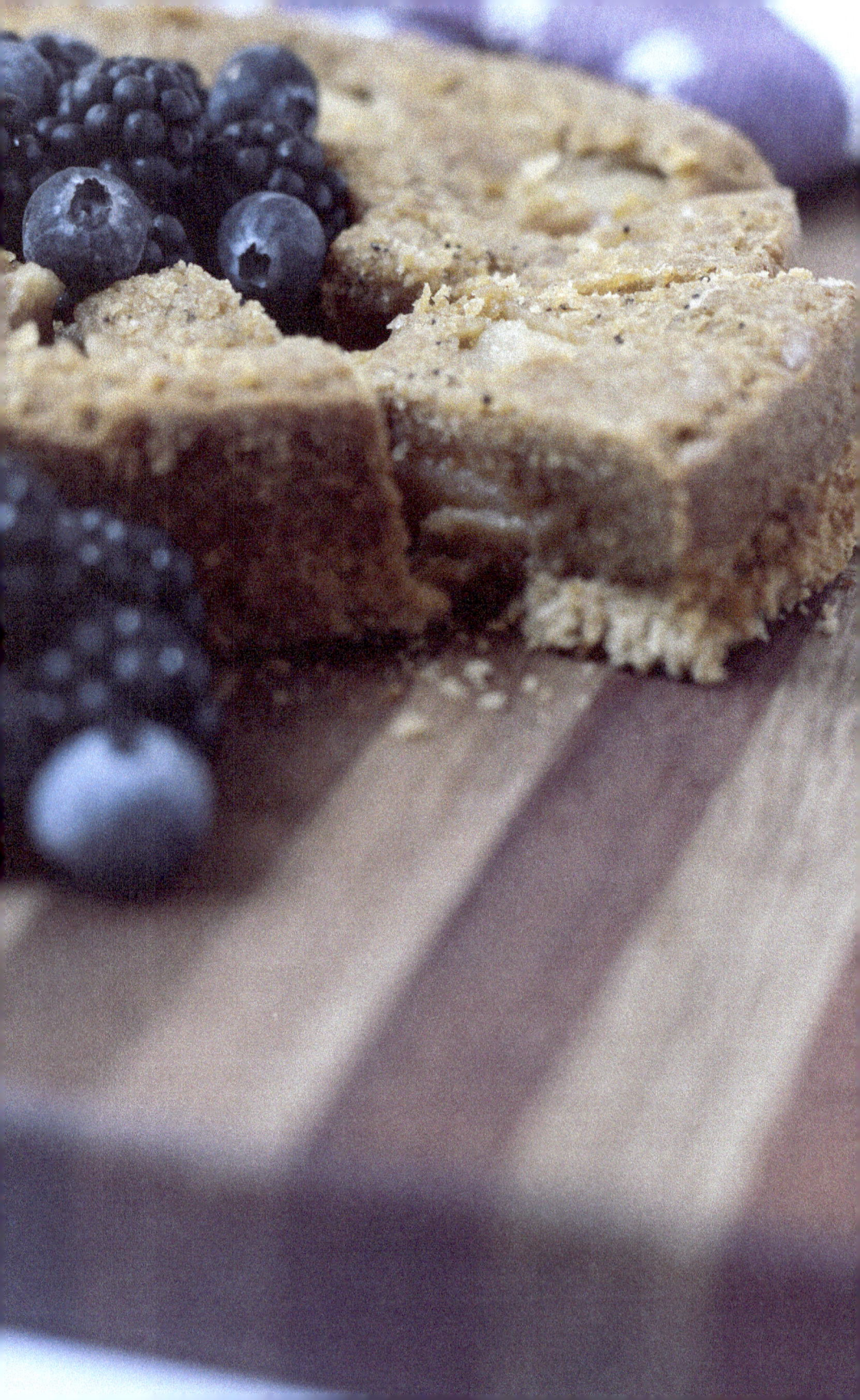

Golden Pear Pudding

This can be served warm as a pudding, but is equally tasty when cooled and served as a cake. Making use of the pears and extract means that it is a fabulous dessert that isn't heavy on sugar.

INGREDIENTS
- 1 700gm (1 lb 9 oz) tin of pears in natural juice
- ¼ cup cornflour
- ¾ cup rice flour
- 2 teaspoon gluten-free baking powder
- ½ cup pear juice extract
- ½ cup rice milk or soya milk
- 2 eggs – separate the yolks and whites
- 1 tablespoon of sunflower oil
- ½ teaspoon nutmeg
- ½ teaspoon cinnamon
- ¼ teaspoon ground cloves

METHOD
1. Pre-heat oven to 160 degrees C)or 320 degrees F).
2. Well grease a pudding dish or individual dishes.
3. Sift all dry ingredients together twice to make the mixture lighter.
4. Mix the oil with the pear juice extract, gradually adding the beaten egg yolks.
5. When mixed, add one third of the flour mixture, fold in one third of the milk and continue adding by thirds until all is mixed.
6. Whisk the egg whites until stiff and fold into the mixture.
7. Cover the bottom of the dish with half the mixture, top with the pear slices (well drained).
8. Pour the remaining other half of the mixture over the pear slices.
9. Bake in a moderate oven for 20 to 25 minutes or until cooked.

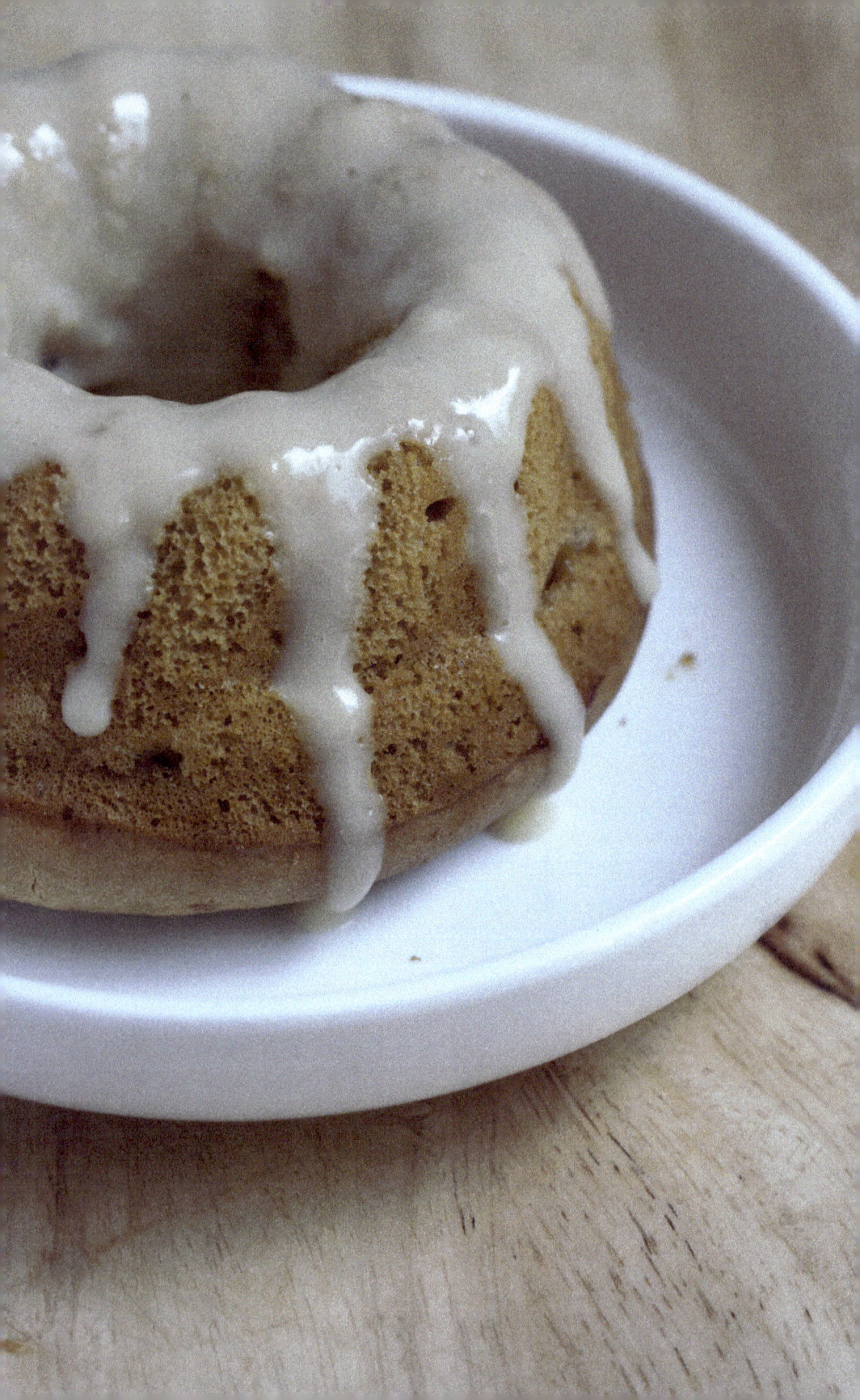

Peach Mango Bake

This was the first dish that my nutritionist OK'd when I was reintroducing a tiny bit of sugar back into my diet. By using the juice in the custard as well, it sweetens the custard without adding extra sugar to the recipe.

INGREDIENTS
Cake:
- 2 cups gluten-free self raising flour
- 2 eggs, lightly beaten
- 1 tablespoon sunflower oil
- ½ cup pear juice concentrate
- 1 tablespoon lemon or lime rind
- 1 tablespoon lemon or lime juice
- ½ cup rice milk
- 700gm (25 oz) tin/jar peaches in mango juice
- 1 teaspoon mixed spice

Custard:
- 2 tablespoons gluten-free custard powder
- 1 cup of mango juice (reserved from tin/jar)
- 1 cup malt-free/sugar-free soy milk or rice milk

METHOD
Cake:
1. Pre-heat oven to 180 degrees C (or 360 degrees F).
2. Lightly grease a pudding dish.
3. Put flour into a bowl and gradually add all the other ingredients except the fruit and mix until smooth.
4. Put half the mixture into the pie dish and spread over the base.
5. Strain the juice from the fruit (save for the custard) and place the stained peaches over the mixture in the pie dish.
6. Pour the remaining mixture over the top of the peaches.
7. Sprinkle mixed spice over the top.
8. Place the pie dish into the oven and bake for 20-25 minutes or until cooked.

Custard:
1. Mix the custard powder with ½ cup of the fruit juice and blend until a smooth paste.
2. Put milk and remaining juice in a small saucepan and heat over medium heat until almost boiling.
3. Add custard mix and stirring constantly bring to the boil.
4. Simmer for 5 minutes.

To serve pour custard over the pudding and top with remaining peaches and sprinkle with mixed spice.

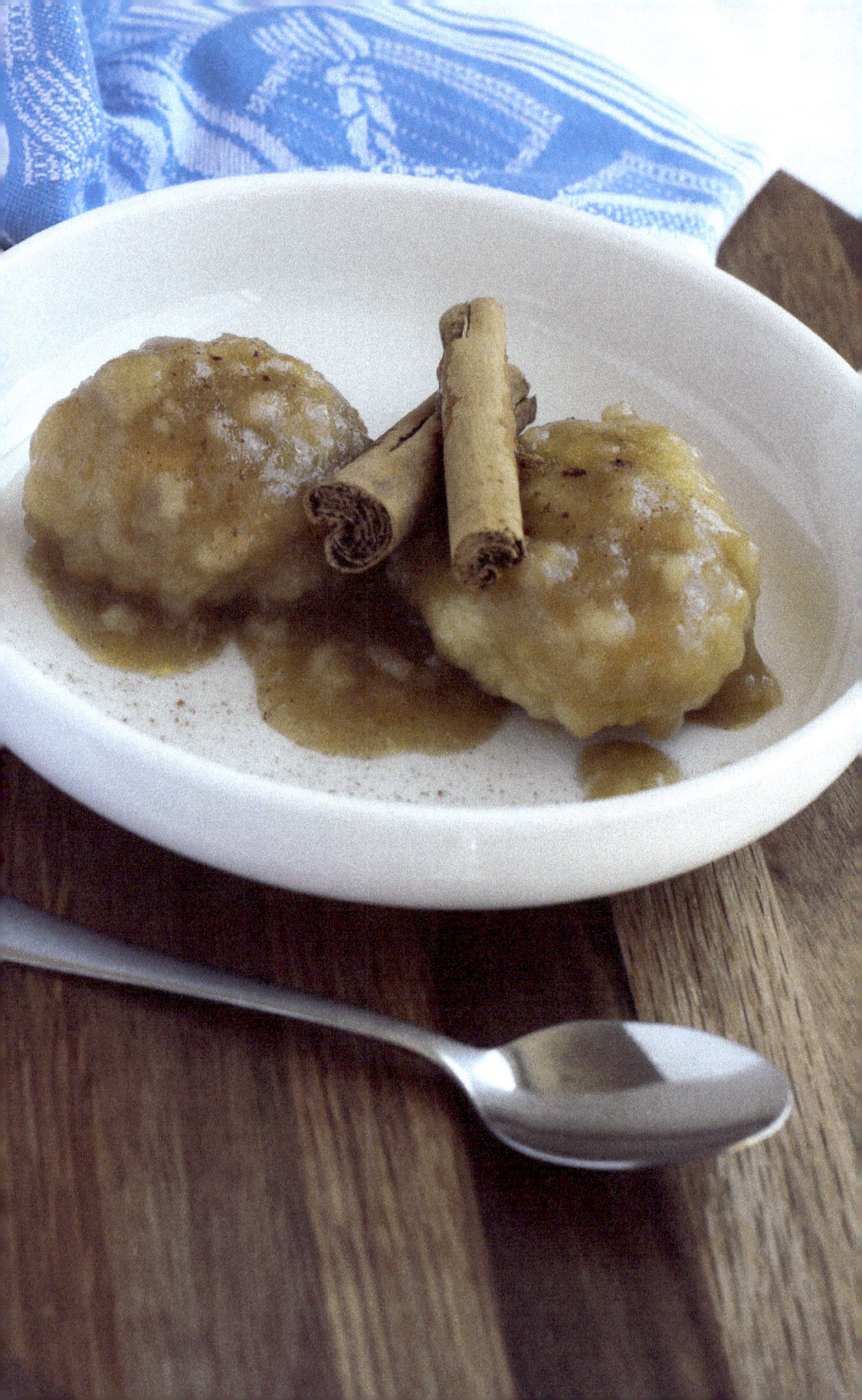

Maple Syrup Dumplings

Golden Syrup Dumplings was a dessert that my family loved so I was keen to create the same dish that was both gluten-free and dairy-free...and by using maple syrup, it has the same yummy flavour with half the sugar of golden syrup!

INGREDIENTS
Dumpling:
- 1 cup gluten-free self raising flour
- 1 tablespoon cold vegan spread, cut into small pieces
- 1 egg, beaten
- 2 tablespoons rice milk

Syrup:
- 2 cups boiling water
- 1 tablespoon vegan spread
- 3 tablespoons pure maple syrup

METHOD
1. Place the flour into a large bowl, rub the vegan spread into the flour with your finger tips, add the egg and milk and with a knife, fat blend into a dough.
2. In a large saucepan add the water, vegan spread and maple syrup.
3. Place the saucepan over high heat and heat the syrup mixture until it comes to the boil, turn down to medium heat.
4. Using two dessert spoons shape the dough into dumpling shapes and drop the dumpling into the hot syrup mixture.
5. Cook the dumplings in the syrup for 20 minutes, turning the dumplings over at 10 minutes.

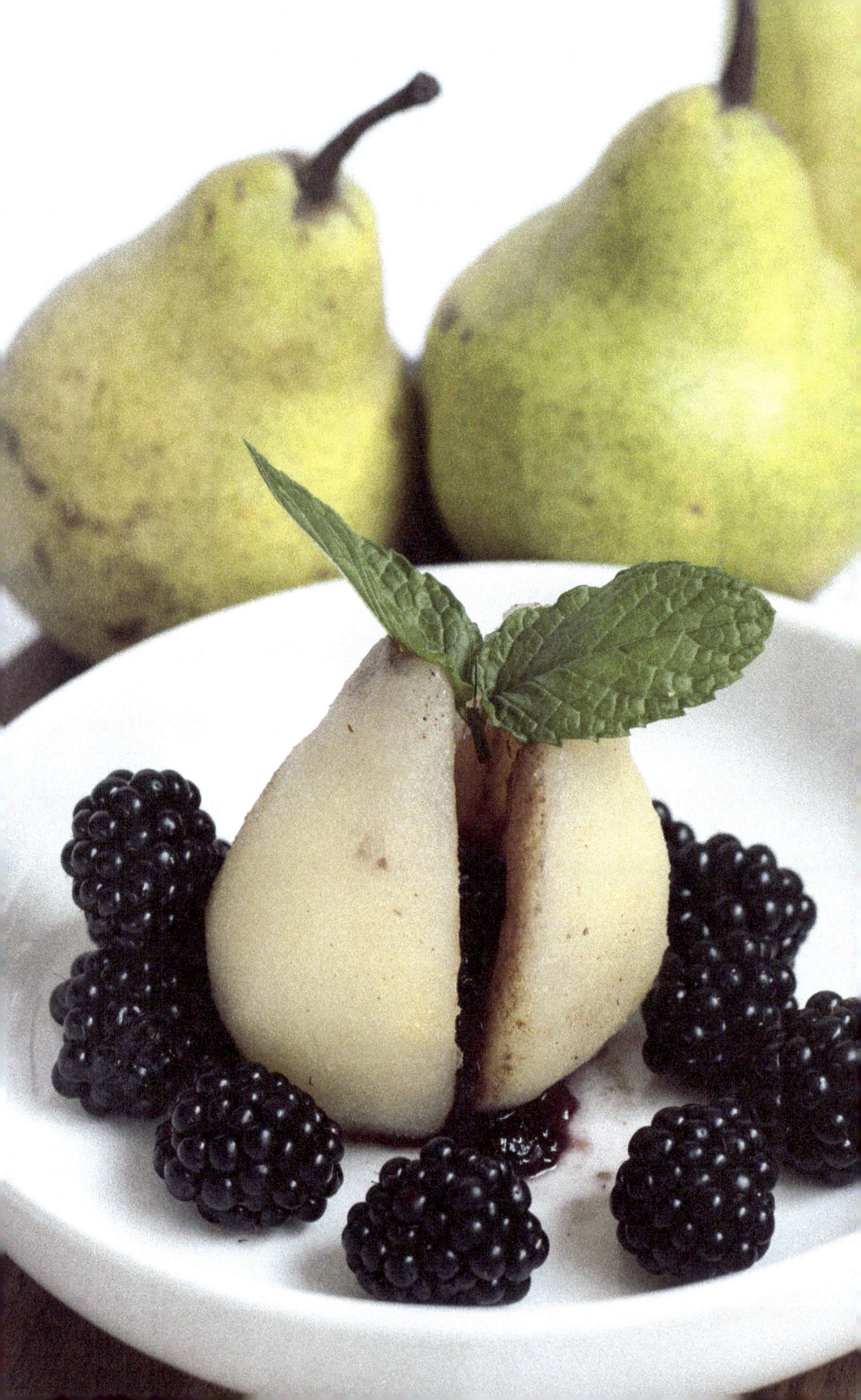

Baked Pear Parcels

These are great if you suddenly have guests and you need to whip up a quick dessert! You can easily store these ingredients in your pantry and this recipe is easy, fast and very tasty.

INGREDIENTS
- Pear, peach or apricot halves (these can be fresh if in season or tinned fruit in natural juices - Allow two halves for each person
- Blueberry jam, all natural and low GI (I use St Dalfour wild blueberry jam)- 1 teaspoon for each parcel
- Vegan spread- ¼ teaspoon for each parcel
- Cinnamon – ¼ teaspoon for each parcel

METHOD
1. Grease large squares of aluminium foil.
2. Place fruit (well drained if tinned), one half facing up, place jam inside, place other half, facing down, on top, sprinkle with cinnamon and wrap tin foil around like a parcel.
3. Place in an ovenproof dish and put in the oven
4. Cook for 15-20 minutes if fresh fruit and 10 minutes if tinned fruit.

Serve with mango gelato (see page 125).

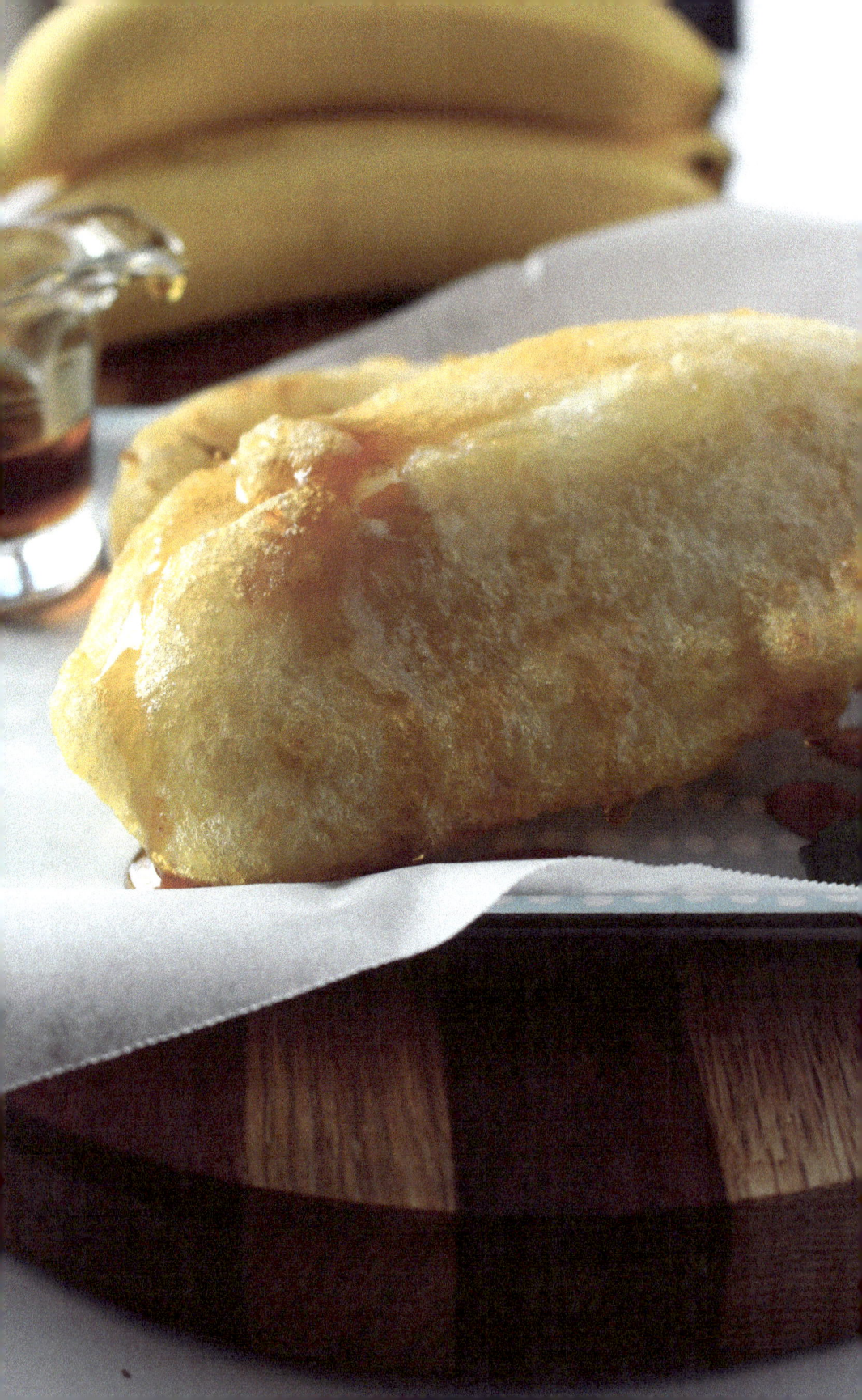

Banana Fritters

A decadent sweet treat and a fond childhood memory is a piece of fruit dipped in batter! Batter, in so many forms, contains both gluten and dairy...so not an ideal dessert these days. However, here is an alternative that is just as simple and just as tasty.

INGREDIENTS
- 1 cup gluten-free self raising flour
- 1 teaspoon baking powder
- 1 cup of cold water (keep in the refrigerator until needed)
- 4 bananas (ripe but firm)
- Extra gluten-free self raising flour (for rolling before battering)
- Oil for frying (I used rice bran oil)

METHOD
1. Sift flour and baking powder into a bowl, then slowly add the cold water and mix to a smooth paste (batter mix).
2. Leave sit for at least 10 minutes.
3. Fill a deep cooker with enough oil to cover the bananas.
4. Bring the oil up to a hot (over medium hot) heat but not smoking.
5. Peel the bananas and roll lightly in the extra flour.
6. Drop the bananas into the batter, letting the excess batter drain back into the bowl.
7. Put the bananas into fry, two at a time to prevent over crowding.
8. Deep fry in the hot oil until golden brown, only takes about two minutes.
9. Remove, drain and place on absorbent paper.
10. Repeat process for the other two bananas.

Delicious served hot with maple syrup and mango gelato (see page 125).

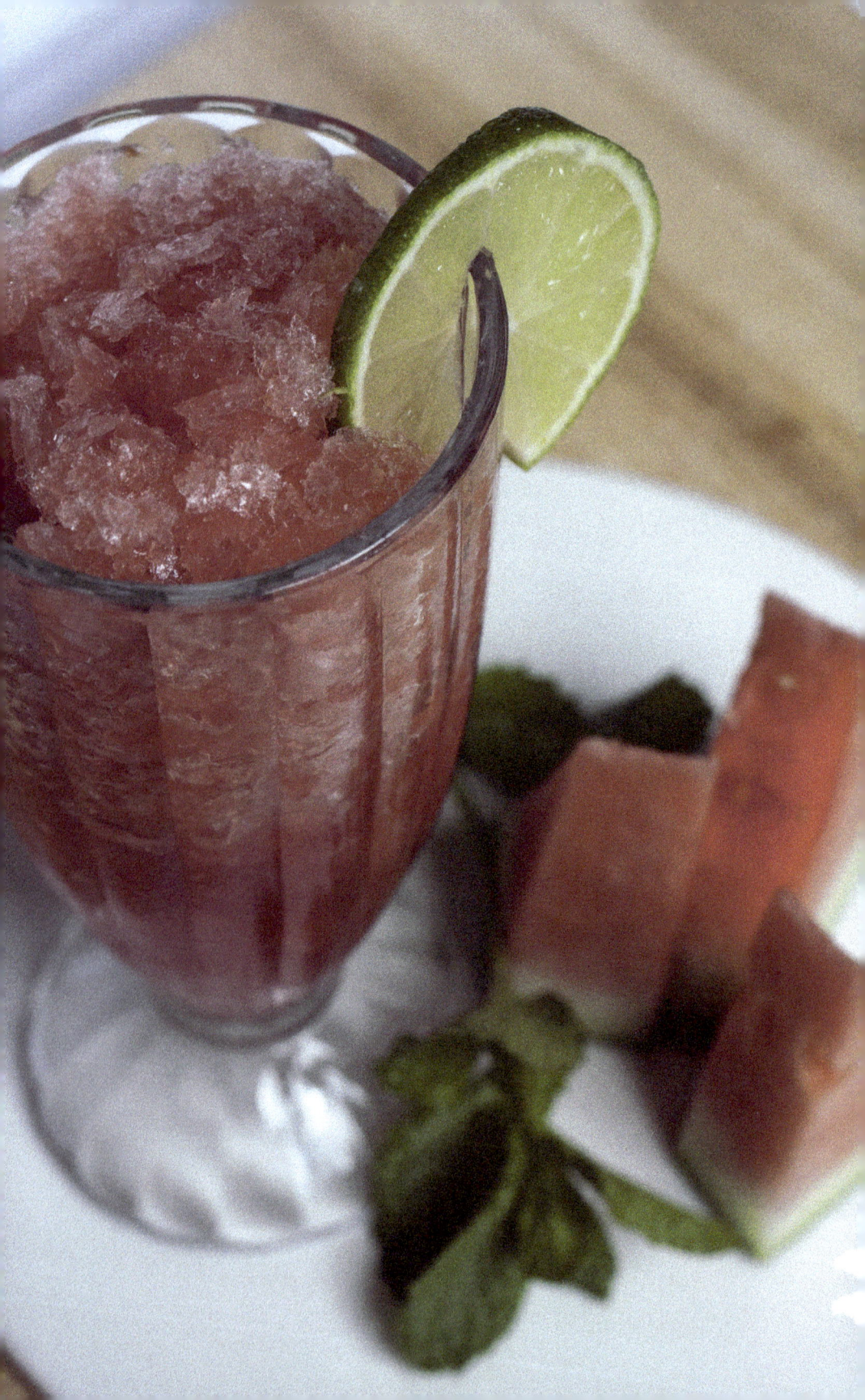

Watermelon Ice

I love this recipe on a hot day! It's very refreshing and cool and it's a lovely dessert when watermelon is in season and not expensive. It's like a healthy, grown up slushy (the grown ups enjoy it as much as the kids do!) and it's ideal after a rich and heavy main course.

INGREDIENTS
- 1kg (2Ibs 3oz) seedless watermelon
- ¼ cup pear juice concentrate
- 1 lemon or lime, use the rind and the juice

METHOD
1. Cut the watermelon into slices, remove skin and cut into pieces.
2. Put watermelon pieces in batches into a blender, and puree.
3. Put puree into a large bowl and slowly add lemon or lime juice, rind and concentrated pear juice, mix well.
4. Pour the mixture into a rigid plastic container and put into the freezer.
5. Freeze uncovered for about 3 hours, or until the mixture is icy and slushy.
6. Turn the mixture into a large bowl and beat to break up ice particles.
7. Return to the plastic container and freeze for a further 2 -3 hours (or until firm).
8. To serve, transfer to the refrigerator and leave for 1 to 1 ½ hours until soft.
9. Mash the ice briefly with a fork and then spoon into parfait dishes.
10. Serve quickly before it melts.

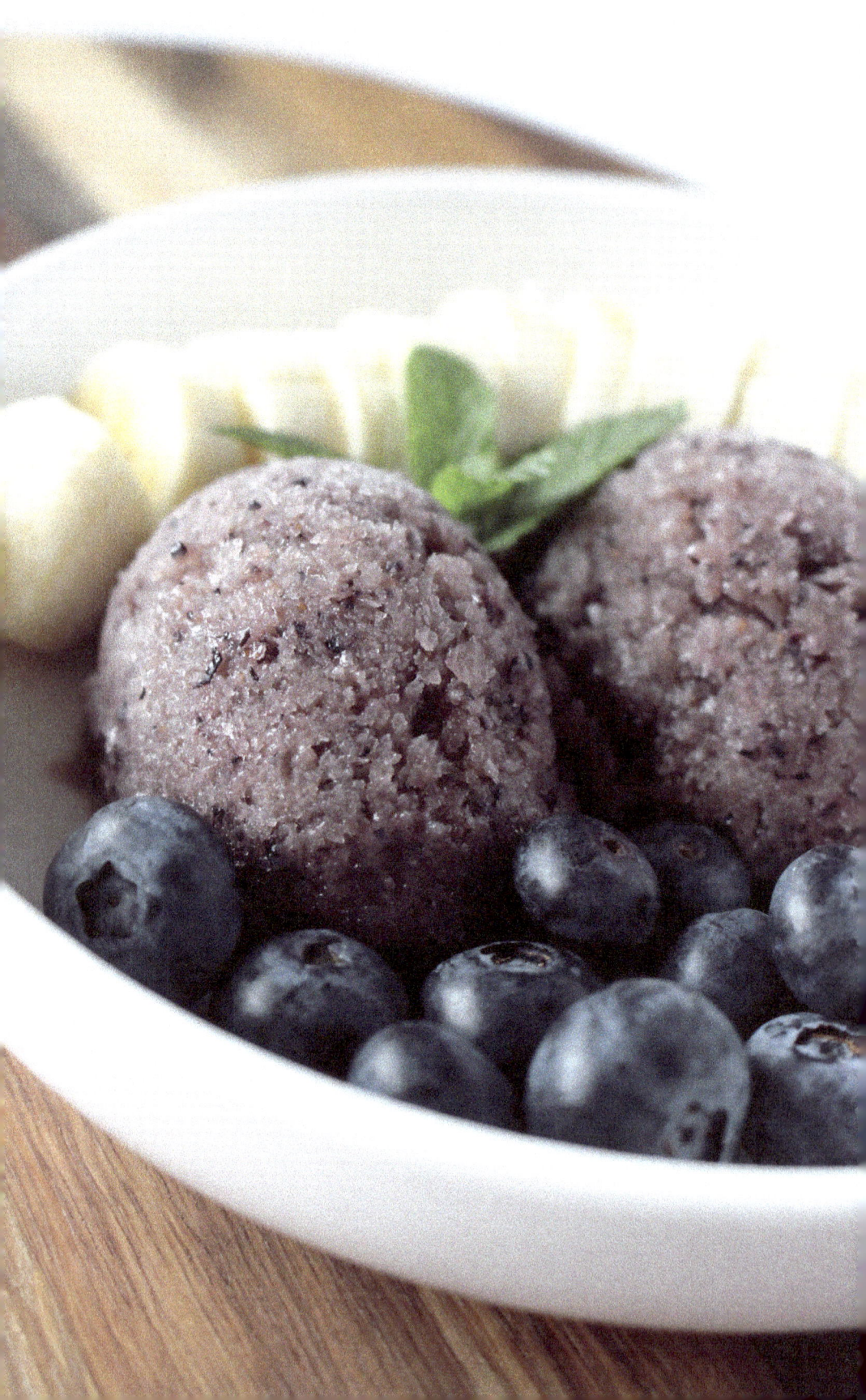

Banana Berry Gelato

You actually don't even need to add the soy yoghurt to this recipe if you don't want - it is just as tasty without it. This is a lovely accompaniment to a hot dessert and it's a great one to keep in your freezer for when you need a little sweet treat.

INGREDIENTS
- 3 ripe bananas
- 1 tablespoon lemon or lime juice
- 1 cup fresh blueberries
- ½ cup vanilla soy yoghurt
- 1 tablespoon maple syrup

METHOD
1. Place peeled bananas and blueberries in a blender and blend until smooth.
2. Add yoghurt, lemon or lime juice and maple syrup and blend until mixture is combined.
3. Put mixture into a large, rigid plastic bowl and place in the freezer until mixture is frozen to a thickness of approximately 2.5cm (1 inch) all the way around the bowl.
4. Remove from freezer and beat the mixture well.
5. Put mixture into a suitable plastic freezer container, cover and return to the freezer until frozen.
6. Remove from freezer and allow to stand until mixture is pliable enough to scoop out.

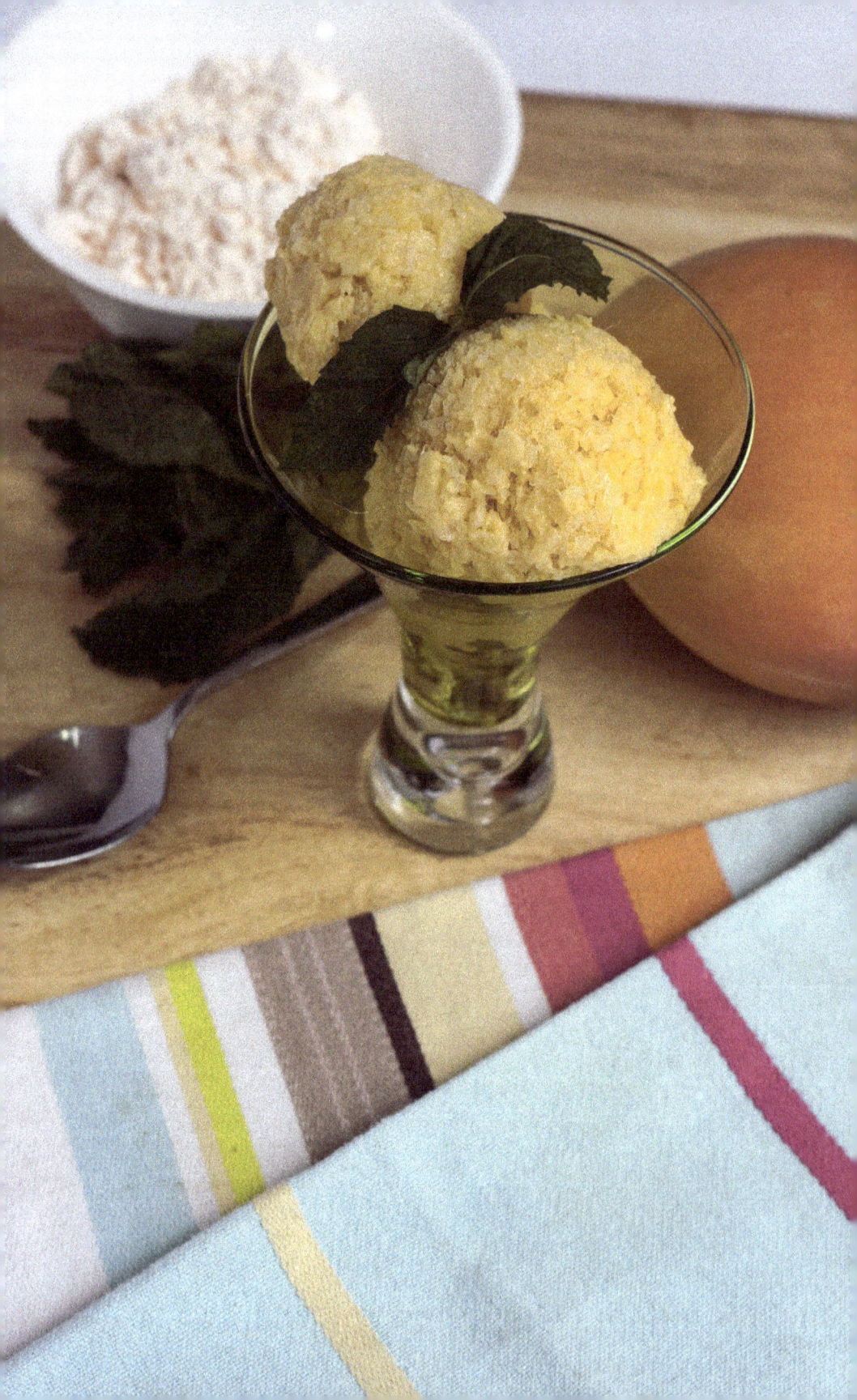

Mango Gelato

This is very refreshing - perfect for a hot day - and it's also a great accompaniment to any baked dessert.

INGREDIENTS
- 2 ripe mangos, peeled and cut into pieces
- 2 tablespoons pure maple syrup
- ½ cup rice milk
- ½ teaspoon vanilla essence

METHOD
1. Place the mangos, maple syrup and vanilla essence into a blender or food processor and blend until smooth.
2. Add the rice milk and blend again.
3. Put the mixture into a rigid plastic container and place in the freezer.
4. Once frozen cover with lid or tin foil.
5. When ready to use leave out for 20 minutes to soften, so you are able to use an ice cream scoop.

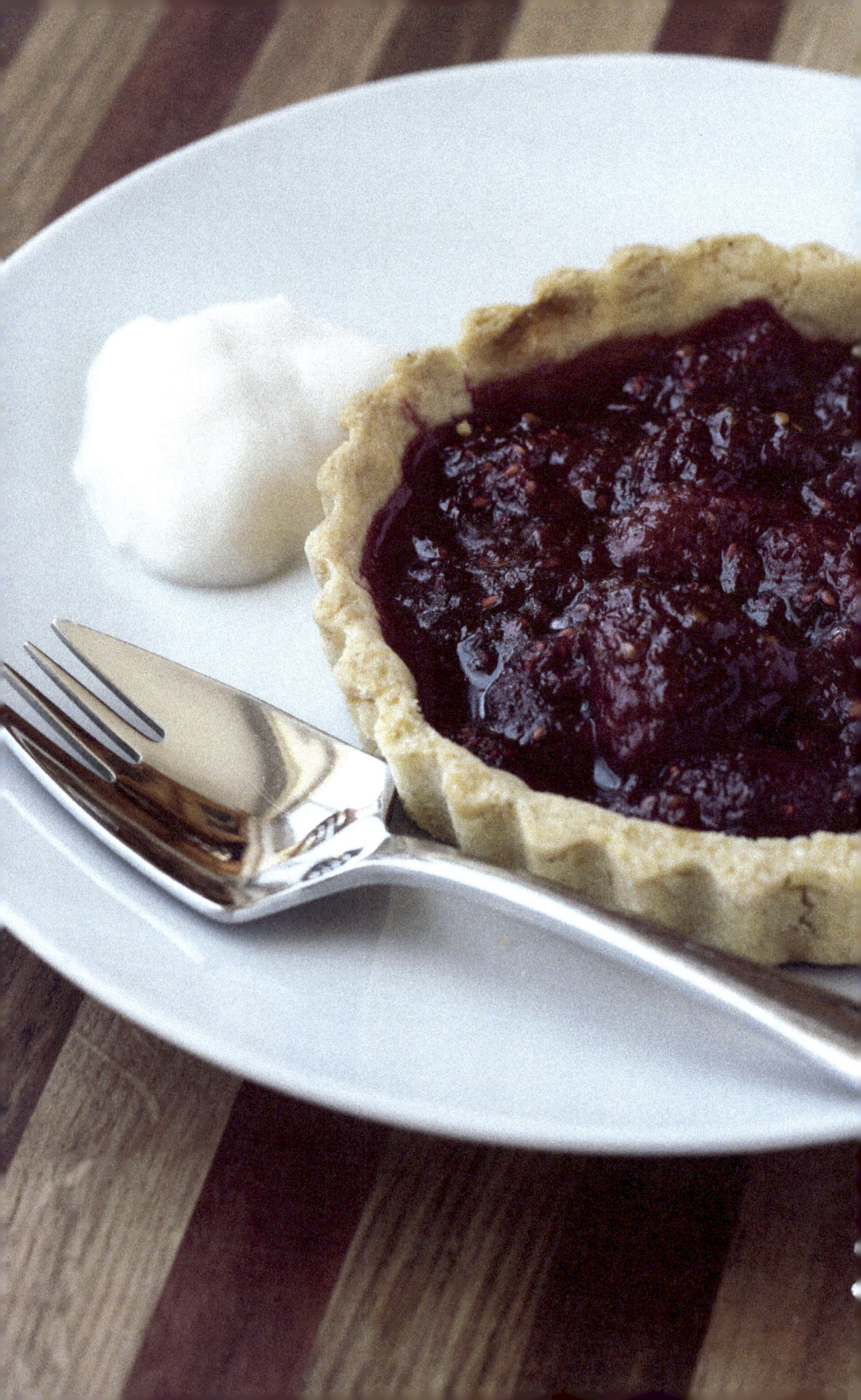

Berry Tart

I enjoy having dinner parties, so it's nice to offer pastries to those who have food restrictions. This dish is delicious, but also very pleasing to the eye when you are dishing it up to guests!

INGREDIENTS
Pastry:
- ¼ cup iced water
- 3 tablespoons vanilla soy yoghurt
- 1 cup gluten-free plain flour
- ½ cup rice flour
- 2 egg yolks
- ¼ teaspoon ground cinnamon
- 100 gm (4 oz) vegan spread (cold from the refrigerator) cut into small pieces

Tart filling:
- 4 cups fresh berries (I used raspberries)
- 2 tablespoons cornflour
- 1 tablespoon lemon or lime juice
- 2 tablespoons all natural, low G.I. berry jam (I use St. Dalfour raspberry jam)

METHOD
1. Pre-heat oven to 180 degrees C or (360 degrees F).

Pastry:
1. Mix the water and yoghurt together, then add the egg yolks and mix together.
2. Sift the flours and cinnamon, rub the small pieces of vegan spread into the mixture with fingertips until the mixture resembles bread crumbs.
3. Gradually add the yoghurt mixture with a knife (fat blend) until the mixture comes together .
4. Gather the dough into a ball and then wrap the dough in plastic wrap and refrigerate for 2 hours.

Tart filling:
1. In a large bowl combine berries, lemon or lime juice and jam.
2. Toss gently until combined.

1. Remove the dough from the refrigerator and cut the dough in half, then into three (six pieces) and shape into six small balls.
2. Roll out gently on lightly floured greaseproof paper and make a 15cm (6 inch) circle and tip into a fluted flan dish, neaten off the edges of excess pastry. Repeat this five more times * As gluten-free pastry breaks easily just press it with your fingers to piece together.
3. Divide the filling evenly among the dishes.
4. Place the dishes into the oven and bake until the filling bubbles and the crust is brown, approximately 15 to 20 minutes.
5. Rest the tarts for 5 minutes then remove from dishes. Serve with vanilla soy yoghurt.

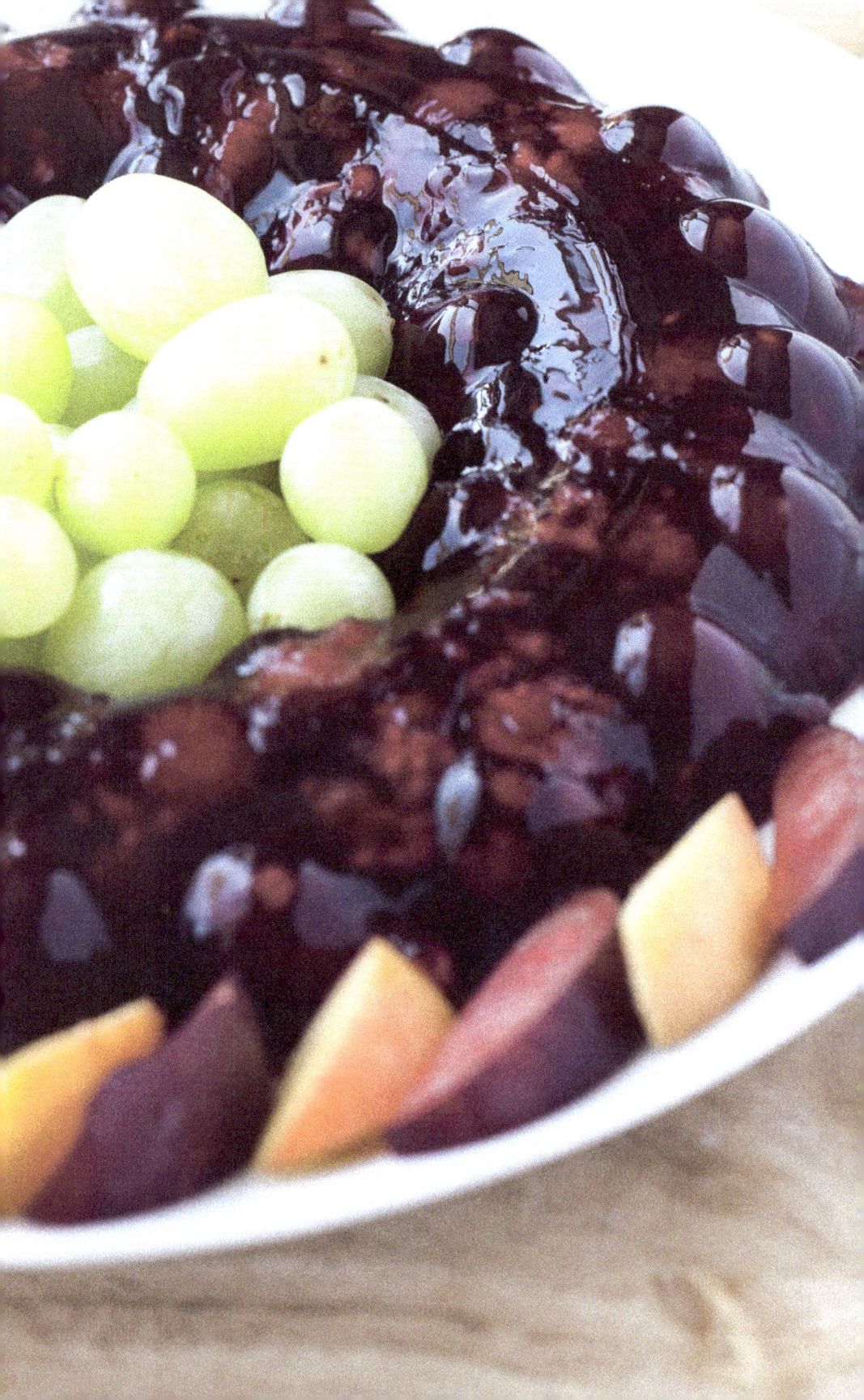

Pomegranate Jelly

Jelly is the perfect summer dessert and this option is a nice healthy alternative to a preservative-filled flavoured jelly.

INGREDIENTS
- 2 cups pomegranate juice
- 1 cinnamon stick
- 1 small orange
- 1 tablespoon powdered gelatine (or vegan equivalent)
- 225gm (8oz) fresh raspberries or berries of your choice
- 1 tablespoon fruit sugar

METHOD
1. Place the pomegranate juice in a saucepan with the cinnamon stick and fruit sugar. Thinly pare the rind from the orange and add that to the saucepan.
2. Heat gently over low heat for 10 minutes, then remove the cinnamon stick and orange peel.
3. Squeeze the juice from the orange into a small dish and sprinkle the gelatine over the top. Leave to swell, then stir into the pomegranate juice to dissolve.
4. Allow to cool until just starting to set, then stir the raspberries into the setting jelly and quickly tip into a four cup mould or serving dish.
5. To turn out, dip the mould quickly into hot water, put a serving plate on top and tip out.

Living With Allergies

Now you know how to cook for yourself and your loved ones, let's talk briefly about life outside your own kitchen and everyday food challenges.

Being diagnosed with food allergies or food intolerances can be a bit of a moment filled with mixed feelings...and it can leave you wondering if life as you know it is over! Don't despair...all you need to do is think ahead.

Eating Out

On one hand, it is great to know why you have been feeling so rubbish. However, it is also really hard to come to terms with realising that all that yummy food you ate before is now off limits. In a way, your eating life flashes before your eyes! No more sharing food with friends and family? No more chocolate topped ice cream at the movies? No more sandwiches and cakes at parties or afternoon tea? Argh!

I didn't want to feel different and I also didn't want to be the downer at every social engagement...the one telling everyone why I couldn't eat this or that. Even worse, once my new diet was on track I felt amazing. I wanted to socialise again and spend time with my family and friends however it felt like every social occasion revolved around food. Food that would make me sick all over again.

I remember being so sick of salad (without the dressing and the croutons, thank you very much) and I quickly started to work out ideas so that I could blend in with everyone and actually eat some regular food.

If I am invited to a fundraiser, or anything that involved 'bringing a plate', I always make sure that I bring along a plate with food that I can eat and that will fill me. I also never leave the house without a herbal tea bag in my purse. A teacup of boiling water and a few pieces of food from the plate that I bring along gets me through without anyone noticing.

If I am at a catered function, I will ask for a mineral water or soda water with a slice of lemon...and ask for it in a wine glass at times! Usually, I can find a tray of sushi with vegetable filling, or a platter with dips and antipasto that has fresh or marinated oiled vegetables on it. I have learnt to enjoy cucumber, carrots, eggplant, sundried tomato and more!

Over time, my handbags have grown in size...I feel a bit like Mary Poppins at times – pulling all sorts of things from the depths of it! I always carry a banana (for the first few years, bananas and pears were the only fruits that I was able to eat, and even though I can eat more of a variety now, they are still my top two!) I also will often carry plain rice crackers; a small bag of pumpkin kernels; sticks of carrot, celery or cucumber; snack packs of natural corn chips or potato chips (make sure they are just sunflower oil and sea salt as other flavours have more additives!) and my trusty herbal tea bags, just in case I go anywhere and there aren't any options.

When people first learn about your food challenges, you might find that you don't get invited to as many places as you once did! Don't take offence, people just don't

know what to feed you.
Over the years, options available when eating out have improved greatly – and the great Paleo trend is helping even more there (although please do double check ingredients, as sometimes they will use certain substitutes that aren't ideal when you have allergies). Most meals on a menu will state if they are Gluten-free (GF), Dairy-free (DF) or Vegetarian (V) but if you have other food problems then don't be embarrassed to ask the waiter to check with the chef. Otherwise, stick to to plain and simple meals such as roast meat and vegetables, grilled meat, fish or poultry without sauces and fresh steamed vegetables or salad. Most restaurants and cafes will have a fresh fruit salad dessert option as well.

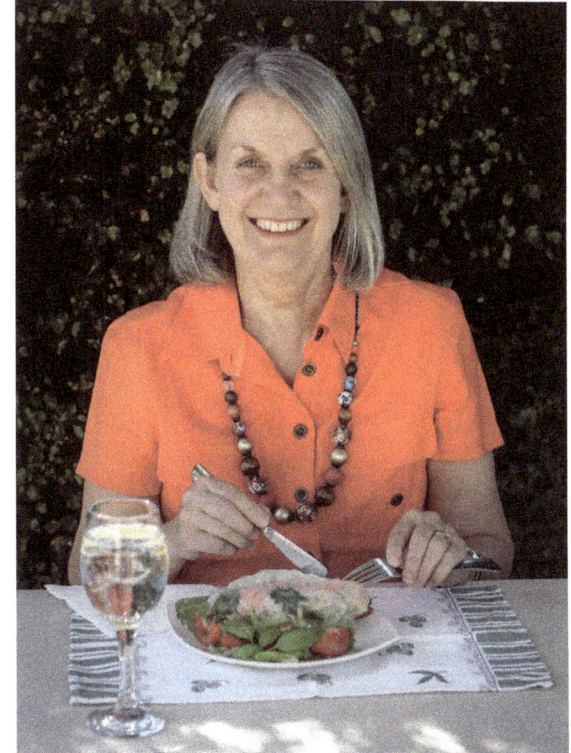

Sticking to your new 'diet' can be hard work – but the benefits are so worth it (not to mention the side effects which can include a trimmer body and more energy!) It will take at least three weeks for your body to get used to your food changes and before you know it, those old foods won't taste as good anyway. I promise!

At Home

Restock your pantry will all your new, basic ingredients as soon as possible. This will mean you are ready to cook, and will have snacks to munch on or take with you. Stock up on gluten-free flours, oils, fruit sugar and fruit syrup, preservative-free dried fruit (if allowed), seeds, spices, herbs, wheat-free soy sauce, pulses and beans, rice, polenta, rice paper sheets and noodles, gluten-free pasta and flakes for cereal such as rice, buckwheat, amaranth and quinoa.

Fill your refrigerator and cupboards with fresh, organic fruit and vegetables and your dairy substitutes.

Remember to read food labels carefully when shopping.

Find ways outside of food to spoil and reward yourself – massage, a yoga or tai chi class, craft or whatever calms you and gives you happiness. We live in a world where, so often, a 'reward' is about 'bad' food. Being diagnosed with an allergy or intolerance is a great excuse to re-train your brain into realising that food is a wonderful way to feel good and fuel your body.

I hope I've helped you see that food can still be a positive and enjoyable part of your world...no matter what! Happy eating!

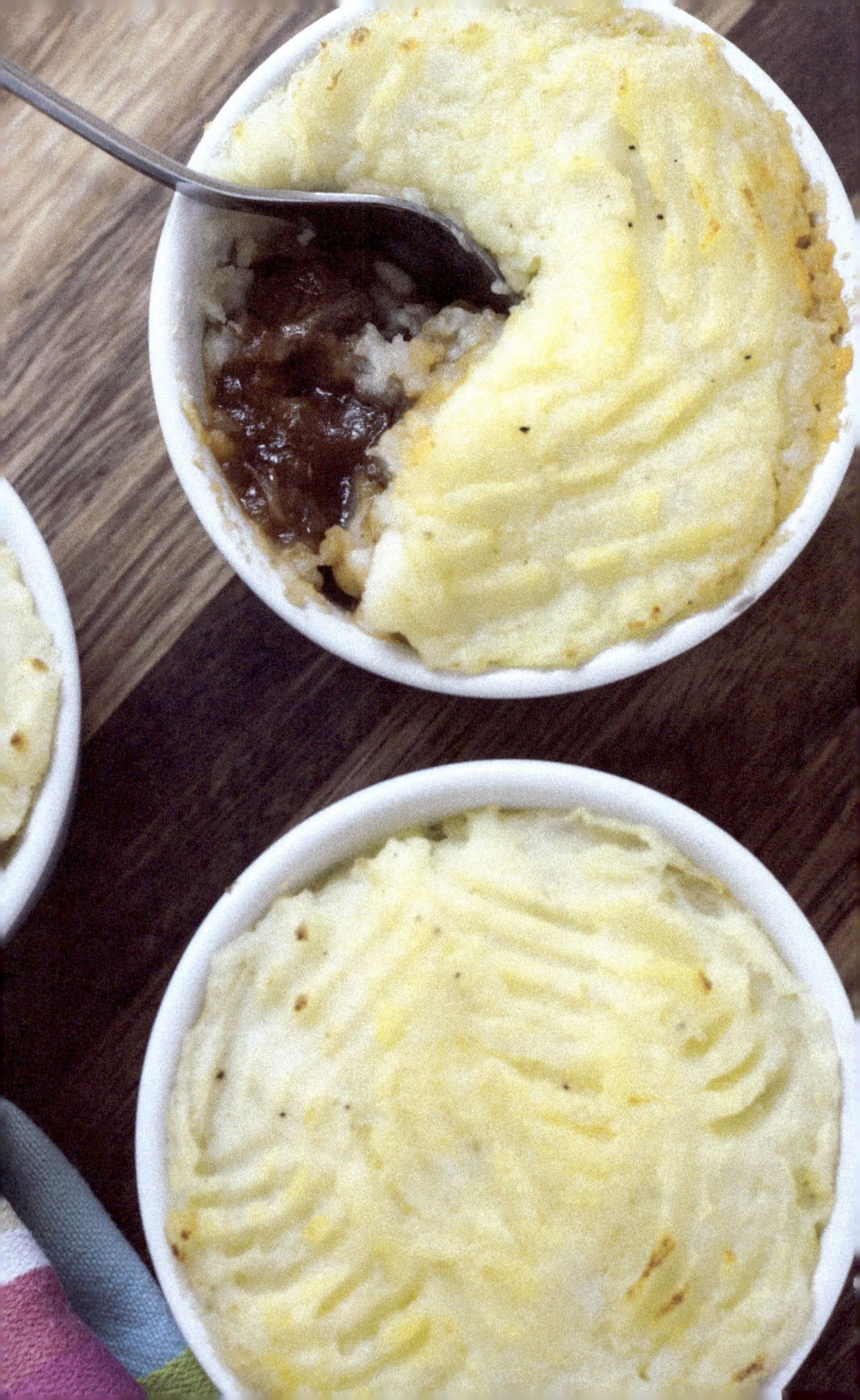

INDEX

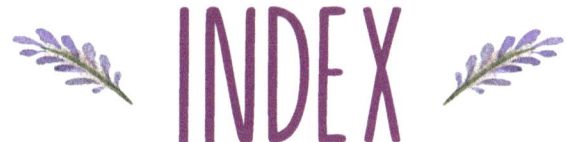

Anchovy, Anchovy & Basil Sauce 33
Anchovy & Basil Sauce 33
Asian Pork 99
Avocado, Avocado Dip 41
Avocado, Corn, Mango & Avocado Salsa 103
Avocado, Fettucine With Tomato & Avocado 89
Avocado Dip 41
Baked Fruit Parcels 117
Banana, Banana & Blueberry Sorbet 123
Banana, Banana Fritters 119
Banana & Blueberry Sorbet 123
Banana Fritters 119
Basil, Anchovy & Basil Sauce 33
Basil, Basil & Sundried Tomato Infused Oil 27
Beef, Beef Goulash 85
Beef, Beef Kebabs 97
Beef, Beef & Potato Pie 87
Beef, Peppered Steaks 101
Beef Goulash 85
Beef Kebabs 97
Beef & Potato Pie 87
Berries, Banana & Blueberry Sorbet 123
Berries, Berry Tarts 127
Berries, Raspberries In Spiced Pomegranate Jelly 129
Berry Tarts 127
Butterfly Pork Steaks With Mustard Sauce & Chives 75
Carrot, Spicy Carrot Soup 53
Chicken, Chicken Kebabs 95
Chicken, Chicken Nuggets 69
Chicken, Chicken Soup 49
Chicken, Chicken Stock 35
Chicken, Lemon Chicken 71
Chicken, Roast Chicken 73
Chicken Nuggets 69
Chicken Soup 49
Chicken Stock 35
Chunky Vegetable & Pork Soup 47
Corn, Mango & Avocado Salsa 103

Crumbed Lamb Chops 81
Dip, Avocado Dip 41
Dip, Hommus 45
Dip, Red Salmon 43
Fettucine With Tomato & Avocado 89
Fish, Red Salmon Dip 43
Fish, Red Salmon Pie 67
Fish, Stuffed Rainbox Trout 63
French Dressing, 29
French Lamb Casserole 79
Fried Rice 59
Fruit Kebabs 107
Garlic, Garlic Infused Oil 25
Garlic, Pork Stir Fry 77
Garlic, Thyme & Garlic Flatbread 57
Garlic Infused Oil, 25
Golden Pear Pudding 111
Herbs, Herbed Oil 23
Herbs, Crumbed Herb Lamb Chops 81
Herbed Oil 23
Hommus Dip 45
Irish Stew 83
Kebabs, Beef Kebabs 97
Kebabs, Chicken Kebabs 95
Kebabs, Fruit Kebabs 107
Kebabs, Lamb Kebabs 96
Lamb, Crumbed Herb Lamb Chops 81
Lamb, French Lamb Casserole 79
Lamb, Irish Stew 83
Lamb, Lamb Kebabs 96
Lamb Kebabs 96
Lemon Chicken 71
Mango, Corn, Mango & Avocado Salsa 103
Mango, Mango Gelato 125
Mango, Peach Mango Bake 113
Mango Gelato 125
Maple Syrup Dumplings 115
Middle Eastern Vegetable Stew 91
Minestrone 51
Mustard, Butterfly Pork Steaks With Mustard Sauce & Chives 75

Mustard, Mustard Sauce 31
Mustard Sauce 31
Oil, Basil & Sundried Tomato Infused Oil 27
Oil, Herbed 23
Oil, Garlic Infused 25
Peach, Peach Mango Bake 113
Pear, Golden Pear Pudding 111
Pear, Baked Pear Parcels 117
Peppered Steaks 101
Pork, Asian Pork 99
Pork, Butterfly Pork Steaks With Mustard Sauce & Chives 75
Pork, Chunky Vegetable & Pork Soup 47
Pork, Garlic & Pork Stir Fry 77
Potato, Beef & Potato Pie 87
Raspberries In Spiced Pomegranate Jelly 129
Red Salmon Dip 43
Red Salmon Pie 67
Roast Chicken 73
Savoury Scones, 55
Scones, Savoury Scones 55
Soup, Chicken Soup 49
Soup, Chunky Vegetable & Pork Soup 47
Soup, Minestrone 51
Soup, Spicy Carrot Soup 53
Spicy Carrot Soup 50
Stock, Chicken Stock 35
Stock, Vegetable Stock 37
Stuffed Rainbow Trout 63
Sun Dried Tomato, Basil & Sundried Tomato Infused Oil 27
Tomato, Fettucine With Tomato & Avocado 89
Tomato, Tomato & Cucumber Salsa 105
Tomato & Cucumber Salsa 105
Thyme & Garlic Flatbread 57
Watermelon Ice 121
Vegetable, Middle Eastern Vegetable Stew 91
Vegetable, Vegetable Stock 37
Vegetable Stock 37

www.ingramcontent.com/pod-product-compliance
Lightning Source LLC
Chambersburg PA
CBHW040335300426
44113CB00021B/2753